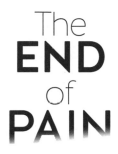

The
END
of
PAIN

The
END
of
PAIN

How **NUTRITION** *and* **DIET**
can **FIGHT CHRONIC**
INFLAMMATORY DISEASE

JACQUELINE LAGACÉ, PhD
with JEAN-YVES DIONNE, BSc Pharm

Foreword by BRYCE WYLDE
Translated by DORINE SOSSO

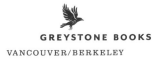
GREYSTONE BOOKS
VANCOUVER/BERKELEY

Greystone Books Ltd.
www.greystonebooks.com

Cataloguing data available from Library and Archives Canada
ISBN 978-1-77164-018-3 (pbk)
ISBN 978-1-77164-019-0 (epub)

Editing by Catherine Plear
Cover and text design by Ingrid Paulson
Illustrations by Jacqueline Lagacé, Paul-André Simard
and Bruno Lamoureux
Printed and bound in Canada by Friesens
Distributed in the U.S. by Publishers Group West

We gratefully acknowledge the financial support of the Canada Council for
the Arts, the British Columbia Arts Council, the Province of British
Columbia through the Book Publishing Tax Credit and the Government of
Canada through the Canada Book Fund for our publishing activities.

Greystone Books is committed to reducing the consumption of old-growth
forests in the books it publishes. This book is one step towards that goal.

TABLE OF CONTENTS

ACKNOWLEDGMENTS / ix
FOREWORD BY BRYCE WYLDE / 1
INTRODUCTION / 5

1 THE ONSET OF PAIN, AND MY SEARCH FOR SOLUTIONS / 11
   1 My experience with chronic pain / 11
   2 Pain in my vertebral column / 12
   3 Arthrosis in my knees / 13
   4 Arthritis/arthrosis in my hands / 15

2 PUTTING THE HYPOTOXIC DIET TO THE TEST / 17
   1 How I discovered Dr. Seignalet's work / 17
   2 The hypotoxic diet: Therapeutic effects
      on the arthritis/arthrosis in my hands / 18
   3 The hypotoxic diet: General effects on my arthritis / 21
   4 Methodological clarifications about this book / 22

3 CLINICAL TESTING AND RESULTS / 24
   1 Who was Dr. Jean Seignalet? / 24
   2 The hypotoxic diet: Theoretical basis and
      practical observations / 31
   3 Diseases that responded positively to the hypotoxic diet / 34
   4 Diseases that responded negatively to the hypotoxic diet / 38

4 KEY ELEMENTS OF DR. SEIGNALET'S DIET / 39

1   Enzymes / 40

2   The importance of small-intestine
integrity in maintaining good health / 43

3   Data from recent medical research confirming
the role of hyper-permeability of the small intestine
in the onset of chronic diseases / 52

4   Dr. Seignalet's nutritional theory and the
contrast between ancient diets and the modern diet / 62

5   Domesticated cereals: A food issue / 65

6   The problem with animal milks / 68

7   Cooking food / 82

8   Update from the latest scientific publications: Links
between "leaky gut," the modern glycotoxin-rich diet
and chronic inflammatory disease / 96

5 BASIC PRINCIPLES OF THE HYPOTOXIC DIET / 100

1   Potential benefits and main requirements / 100

2   Analysis of various foods / 103

3   How I adapted to the hypotoxic diet / 107

**6 MAINTAINING A PROPER PHYSIOLOGICAL BALANCE:
PRODUCTS, PRINCIPLES AND INFORMATION / 112**

1   Soy and human health / 112

2   Mineral waters / 114

3   Balance between alkalinity and acidity in body fluids / 115

4   Probiotics / 116

5   Reduction of micronutrients (vitamins, mineral salts
and trace elements) in foods cultivated during the last
seven decades / 119

6   Vitamin and mineral supplements / 123

7   Can chondroitin sulfate and glucosamine sulfate
reduce arthrosis symptoms? / 128

8   Essential fatty acids, saturated fats and trans fats / 129

9   Effects of sugars, especially fructose, on hypertension,
diabetes types 1 and 2 and kidney function / 133

**7   THE IMMUNE SYSTEM'S STRATEGIES IN CHRONIC
INFLAMMATORY DISEASES / 137**
1   Inflammatory responses / 137
2   Acute inflammatory response / 139
3   Chronic inflammatory response / 140
4   Tolerance and autoimmunity / 142
5   The role of HLA molecules in the immune response / 144
6   Autoimmune diseases / 145
7   Some examples of autoimmune diseases linked
     to different types of HLA / 147

8   RHEUMATOID ARTHRITIS AND THE HYPOTOXIC DIET / 148
1   A typical autoimmune disease: Rheumatoid arthritis / 148
2   Review of recent scientific literature on the role of
     genetic factors and the environment in the development
     and persistence of rheumatoid arthritis / 160

**9   OTHER AUTOIMMUNE DISEASES THAT RESPONDED
POSITIVELY TO THE HYPOTOXIC DIET / 168**
1   Ankylosing spondylitis: Hypotheses and results / 168
2   Multiple sclerosis: Hypotheses and results / 170

**10   SEIGNALET'S THEORY ON THE PHENOMENON OF TISSUE
DEPOSITION AS THE CAUSE OF CERTAIN CHRONIC
INFLAMMATORY DISEASES / 173**
1   The deposition theory: The role of intestinal wastes / 173
2   Osteoarthritis—A disease resulting from deposit
     formation in tissues: Characteristics and pathogenesis / 176
3   Fibromyalgia / 181
4   Type 2 or non-insulin-dependent diabetes / 182

11   DISEASES OF ELIMINATION / 186
1   Seignalet's theory of diseases of elimination / 186
2   Colitis or irritable bowel syndrome / 187
3   Crohn's disease / 188
4   Acne: A skin pathology involving excretion / 189
5   Atopic eczema (also called atopic dermatitis) / 190
6   Asthma / 190

12 DRUGS USED TO TREAT INFLAMMATORY DISEASE / 193

1   Anti-inflammatory drugs: Generalities and
modes of action / 193

2   The major classes of painkillers / 195

3   Side effects of NSAIDS / 198

**13 ATTEMPTS TO EXPLAIN THE LACK OF CONSENSUS ON
USING TARGETED NUTRITION TO PREVENT AND TREAT
MANY CHRONIC DISEASES (DESPITE THE PUBLICATION
OF NUMEROUS CONVINCING STUDIES) / 201**

1   Other opposition to nutritional change / 202

2   Why is it difficult and even threatening for healthcare
professionals to be using diet as a treatment
for chronic diseases? / 203

3   Methods of subsidy distribution for government
research / 205

4   Pharmaceutical companies' grip on healthcare / 206

5   Marketing and R&D: impact on medicine / 207

6   Non-recommended use of drugs and insufficient
study of drug side effects / 208

EPILOGUE / 210

GLOSSARY / 217

ENDNOTES / 225

REFERENCES FOR THE FOREWORD / 265

APPENDIXES / 267

INDEX / 276

ACKNOWLEDGMENTS

I am extremely grateful to everyone at Éditions Fides Inc. for their recognition of the importance of this message and for their tireless work, which has greatly contributed to the significant success of the French version of my book. I have appreciated that this project has brought us our friendship. Thanks also to Dorine Sosso for translating my book into English.

Thank you to those responsible at Greystone Books who believed in the importance of making this message available to an English-speaking readership. A special thanks to Catherine Plear, my editor, for making sure the message remains clear, smooth and practical. Your talented editorial genius made this such a better book, through all its iterations. Thanks also to Bryce Wylde for agreeing to write the foreword to this book and Andrea Damiani, for her marketing work.

I would like to express my special gratitude to my husband, Hubert; my children, Magali and Paul-André Simard, who have always encouraged and supported me on this journey; and to my son-in-law, Alain Dubois, for making my website come alive.

To Hubert, for his unfailing love and support.

Also to my daughter, Magali Simard, and to my son, Paul-André Simard, for their courage and creativity.

FOREWORD

Pain is the most common reason individuals seek medical attention. It is an unpleasant sensory experience associated with damage to body tissues, organs, bones or muscles, or even an unpleasant emotional experience related to psychological trauma. But the number of people who experience chronic pain of one kind or another will shock you: more than 100 million in North America alone. What's more, 40 million of these people do not respond to over-the-counter pain medication. According to the National Institutes of Health, the annual cost of chronic pain in the United States, including health-care expenses, lost income and lost productivity, is estimated to be about $100 billion. These numbers are all staggering, and as the population ages, all of these estimates are expected to grow rapidly.

Pain is not a disease; it is a symptom. It is the body's crucial signal to us: "Houston, we have a problem." You can't ignore it. Designed to catch your attention, pain is indeed one of those things that almost everyone is inclined to look into. Interestingly, most people have pain that cannot be traced to a cause such as fracture, infection, cancer, or significant changes that show up in tests or on imaging studies like MRIS and CT scans. When you experience pain, the real issue becomes what course you'll follow if your pain is not rapidly resolved. Most people who are "in it" understandably look for a quick fix and may not realize that diet may be a major contributing, underlying and even causative factor in their pain.

"If you want to feel better and lead a healthier life, plus lose some weight and reduce your pain, then stop eating fast food." If your doctor offers up this age-old rhetoric, please excuse him or her. While it is obviously relevant advice, it is also antiquated. Probably the last things you or your doctor would ever suspect of contributing to your arthritis pain are the fiber-rich whole-grain bread you've eaten all your life, the "prescribed" glass of milk that you're proud to drink daily or just *how* you've been cooking your fish. This is all *healthy,* right?

When it comes to conventional pain management, the mainstream solution has too narrowly focused on the use of analgesics such as acetaminophen, oxycodone, propoxyphene or nonsteroidal anti-inflammatory drugs (NSAIDs) such as aspirin, Advil and ibuprofen. It may come as a big surprise that most of these treatments have actually shown limited effectiveness in randomized controlled clinical trials or are known to have significant and often severe side effects. These drugs may be effective for use in the short term, but they are the leading cause of death due to drugs! To avoid the cardiac risks and the gastrointestinal and dependency issues associated with traditional pain treatments (and particularly with long-term use), many people have turned to complementary and alternative medicines (CAMs) such as dietary supplements.

But what if you could put an end to your pain by using an approach that may prove more effective than drugs and more natural than dietary supplements, and which is also impeccably safe? *The End of Pain* makes a solid case that many of our modern-day foods are toxic because they are vastly different from the foods eaten by our ancestors. This book proceeds from the premise that the human digestive system has not had time to adapt to these changes and that cooking at high temperatures can modify the protein structure of foods, all of which contribute to creating a state in which the body begins to attack itself. Jacqueline Lagacé has brilliantly shed light on the fact that pain may be better addressed by consciously *removing* triggers from your diet rather than relying on pills. Having experienced significant pain herself, Jacqueline draws on her skills as a seasoned researcher, and in a been-there-done-that manner, masterfully integrates the work of the French clinician and professor Dr. Jean Signalet—whose life work was relating autoimmune diseases to the modern diet. Lagacé explains exactly how you can employ optimal nutrition, the hypotoxic diet and other nutritional techniques to fight chronic inflammatory disease.

If we really are what we eat, then consuming mostly non-modified foods that can be more completely digested, assimilated, and used properly by the body, and also accepted by the immune system, may very well end up becoming the end of *your* pain.

Bryce Wylde, BSC, DHMHS, RNC
Alternative health expert and host of *Wylde on Health*

INTRODUCTION

WHY DID I WRITE THIS BOOK?

I wrote this book primarily to inform those suffering from chronic pain that dietary changes can put an end to their pain and give them a quality of life that they never thought possible. The dietary changes recommended in this book are the results of the observations, thoughts and experiments of researchers and doctors who are not afraid to challenge certain dietary traditions: those that are considered healthy but which, in the long run, harm a significant number of people.

I became interested in how nutrition therapy could treat chronic inflammatory disease and its associated pain through the work of Dr. Jean Seignalet. Dr. Seignalet was a French clinician and medical researcher, as well as a specialist in immunology, rheumatology, gastroenterology and nutrition therapy. After having worked as a researcher and having practiced medicine for about twenty years, Dr. Seignalet reoriented his research and medical practice towards nutrition therapy because conventional medicine was unable to efficiently and sustainably help patients affected by chronic inflammatory disease. He dedicated the last eighteen years of his medical-research career to developing a nutritional method that could fight chronic pain and control the progress of many inflammatory diseases. He used the knowledge he gained from researching nutrition therapy to treat more than 2,500 patients affected by chronic pain associated with diverse inflammatory diseases. Of the 115 inflammatory diseases that he treated with his diet, 91 responded positively in about 80 percent of the patients who followed the diet correctly. He also observed a remission of disease and, in general, a total disappearance of pain in a great majority of patients. In addition, in cases in which the affected tissues had not been permanently destroyed by inflammatory processes, patients who were successfully treated gradually regained lost functionalities in the short or long term. Such results are ignored or denied by the vast majority of health professionals, who continue to believe that a change in diet cannot control an inflammatory disease and its associated chronic pain.

Despite my own definite skepticism and the negativity of some doctors, I found that by following Dr. Jean Seignalet's basic principles of nutrition, I was able to put an end to my severe, uncontrollable chronic pain from the osteoarthritis in my spine and the arthritis in my hands.

I had a number of reasons for trying the Seignalet diet:

1) Conventional medicine completely failed for me.
2) I was exasperated by unbearable chronic pain, from which I could find no respite.
3) The scientific arguments of Dr. Seignalet seemed plausible to me, given my own training and research experience in microbiology and immunology.
4) Dr. Seignalet's surprising success, recorded over a period of eighteen years, involving about 2,500 patients affected by chronic inflammatory disease, seemed very real.

5) On a daily basis, I was consuming large quantities of the two food types considered cofactors in triggering chronic inflammatory disease in those who have a genetic predisposition.

6) It seemed possible to quickly verify the effects of the diet, as the author confirmed that significant improvements usually began about three months after starting the diet.

7) Given the intensity of the pain I had in my hands, I had nothing to lose. Rather than take medication, I preferred to try a diet that presented no side effects.

8) Finally, as a researcher, I was curious, and that definitely played a role in my decision.

I must mention that my expectations were very modest. In the best-case scenario, I hoped for a reasonable reduction in the pain in my hands. I never thought it possible to recover the normal use of my hands, and I was not expecting any results concerning other health problems (which I'll discuss later). The surprise came when I noticed, after just ten days of being on the diet, that the pain in my hands had completely disappeared. Even more surprising was the fact that just three months after I started the diet, one after the other, I was able to gradually bend the different joints in my hands, which I had previously been unable to do. This progress, accomplished over a period of about sixteen months, was accompanied by the gradual disappearance of the sensitivity I used to feel when I applied pressure to my finger joints. I should emphasize that these results were obtained without any practical exercises to relax my finger joints. I generally became aware of the additional progress made during my morning stretches, as I noticed I was now able to move a particular joint. I was also surprised, after being on the Seignalet diet for more than a year, by a noticeable improvement in my knee joints and in my spine. They had been affected by symptomatic arthritis for three years and twenty years, respectively.

Because I had experienced such exceptional personal results as a result of following Dr. Seignalet's diet, I would frequently talk about it whenever I had the opportunity. I discovered that Dr. Seignalet's work was virtually unknown outside France. Up until 2010, I never met anyone, not even in the health sector, who knew about it. Yet his work mostly focused on arthritis, a disease that affects the majority of individuals at one point or another. In fact, arthritis encompasses hundreds of different conditions, of which the best known are rheumatoid arthritis, osteoarthritis, fibromyalgia, gout, lupus erythematosis, scleroderma, ankylosing spondylitis and carpal tunnel syndrome, just to name the most common (see www.arthitis.ca).[1] Generally, the pathology of all these diseases involves chronic inflammation. Even arthrosis, often described as noninflammatory arthritis, also presents a non-negligible inflammatory process, according to recent studies.[2] The causes of arthritis are unknown, and current conventional treatment methods cannot cure it. In fact, the medications used now focus mainly on reducing pain and slowing the disease's progress, which they do with relatively modest success.

With all this in mind, I deemed it very important to make Dr. Seignalet's work known in Quebec. I decided to describe my personal experience with arthritis in this work and to popularize Dr. Seignalet's teachings, which are described in the last edition of his book, published in 2004,[3] *L'Alimentation ou la troisième médecine*. This 600-page book is not readily accessible to the general public because of the level of language it uses: for those with no medical training, it's very difficult to understand. Yet it is crucial to insist on the basic concepts of the Seignalet diet because a good understanding of the scientific principles behind this diet can provide the motivation to follow it, especially as it's a long-term diet that imposes major changes on normal and accepted eating habits.

Thus, I wrote this book to make Dr. Seignalet's teachings available to the general public. I carried out an exhaustive literature review of recent scientific material in order to keep abreast of all the new and recent theories on nutrition and also those related to chronic inflammatory diseases. My goal was to find out if other research projects could explain, complement, validate or invalidate the main elements of Dr. Seignalet's theories. Based on this literature review, I tried to include complementary information on controversial topics such as the consumption of soybeans, mineral water and probiotics, the presence of micronutrients in foods from industrial agriculture, and the intake of vitamins and mineral supplements, chondroitin sulfate, glucosamine, etc. This review (conducted using the PubMed, Medline and Google Scholar medical databases) made it possible for me to highlight and compare the similarities and differences between Dr. Seignalet's theories and theories from nutrition-related fields on degenerative and chronic inflammatory diseases. Finally, my twenty-five years of experience in biomedical research, of which seventeen have been spent as a research professor and director of a microbiology and immunology laboratory at a university, greatly contributed to my decision to publish this work.

I hope that the information in this volume will help many people suffering from chronic inflammatory disease significantly improve their quality of life. I would also like to see health professionals who specialize in the treatment of chronic inflammatory diseases and pain become aware that a *targeted diet* can fight these conditions.

1

THE ONSET OF PAIN, AND MY SEARCH FOR SOLUTIONS

1. MY EXPERIENCE WITH CHRONIC PAIN

In my introduction to this book, I emphasized the arthritis I had in my hands because it caused me the most pain and most affected my quality of life. This condition drove me to nutrition therapy in search of relief, as traditional medicine and alternative medicine such as acupuncture, osteopathy, physiotherapy and kinesitherapy had failed to bring any notable relief to the chronic pain in my hands. Even though I was greatly afflicted by the loss of the normal use of my hands, it was the sharp, virtually constant pain that was the most unbearable. This illness, which presented symptoms of both rheumatoid arthritis and arthrosis, had, between 2004 and 2007, turned me into an insomniac, to the point of affecting my quality of life. To present an overall picture of the effects of Dr. Seignalet's diet on my quality of life as a whole, I will provide a detailed description here of the various symptoms of my arthritis/arthrosis.

2. PAIN IN MY VERTEBRAL COLUMN

Like many others, I periodically suffered from back pain in the region of the fifth lumbar vertebra. It began when I turned thirty, after I was involved in a collision of bumper cars in an amusement park. At the instant of the impact, I felt pain in my lower back, which became localized for two or three weeks around the sciatic nerve located in the gluteus and the left thigh. The pain gradually faded, even though from time to time I would feel it in the lumbar area. It was bearable and temporary, and aspirin would make it disappear.

When I was about forty-five years old, the painful episodes became more frequent and more acute. Sometimes, just straightening as I stood up would result in extreme pain. I consulted with physicians, who diagnosed arthrosis and recommended aspirin or Tylenol and physiotherapy to reduce the pain and inflammation. I followed some physiotherapy treatments, but with no great results. Later on, an acquaintance told me about a physiotherapist who specialized in osteopathy and who had successfully treated him for a serious and extremely painful lumbar condition. For many years, I worked with this physiotherapist during my most acute episodes of pain, and I must acknowledge that these treatments truly helped me. In addition, every morning when I woke up, I did a series of exercises prescribed by this therapist. These exercises both toned and strengthened the muscles around my vertebral column and helped me prevent a relapse. Most of the time, I had no trouble with my back as long as I did my exercises in the morning and avoided putting too much pressure on my lumbar spine as I went about my daily activities. My back problem was definitely under control, and I only suffered two or three serious crises a year.

In my early fifties, I started feeling acute pain in my neck that often radiated towards the left shoulder. X-rays revealed the presence of arthrosis. Osteopathic, acupuncture and kinesitherapy treatments generally provided me with relief for a few months. However, since the end of 2008—a year and a half after I started the hypotoxic diet—I no longer suffer from cervical (neck) pain.

When I started Dr. Seignalet's diet on June 10, 2007, in a bid to treat the arthritis/arthrosis in my hands, I had no expectations regarding the other joint diseases I suffered. In spring 2008, about one year after starting the diet, I noticed that I no longer felt the least lumbar pain when I got up in the morning, which was very unusual. I then gave in to laziness as I had lost motivation, and slowly stopped the daily exercises for my back. I even began to get careless, going as far as wielding a shovel in my garden and shoveling snow. After falling in January 2009, I had to acknowledge that even though the state of my lumbar column had greatly improved, I still needed to do the exercises for my back every morning.

Now, it is obvious that even though it stopped the progression of arthrosis in my lumbar region and strengthened my spine, the Seignalet diet did not repair everything in my vertebral joints. However, I can confirm that there has been a 90 percent improvement, to say the least. I no longer suffer from pain in my lower back—except in very rare situations when I go overboard and when I get up after a long meal or movie—and I no longer have any trouble straightening up as I used to.

3. ARTHROSIS IN MY KNEES

In the fall of 2004, I started feeling some stiffness and pain in both knees, especially in the left knee. At the beginning of 2006, I bought a treadmill, planning to systematically walk for about fifteen minutes daily, depending on how much I could tolerate at any given time. At first, as I did these exercises, I would feel an itchy sensation and pain that was sometimes severe or light depending on the day. During the winter of 2006–07, I had to wear elastic knee braces, as my knees had lost their strength and hurt during and after skiing.

In May 2007, as I walked off a plane after a very long flight, I felt a round lump in the back of my left knee. This lump made it impossible for me to fully stretch out my leg and made walking difficult and painful, even though most of the time the pain did not disturb me that much. The general practitioner I consulted requested a venous Doppler ultrasound of my lower limbs that revealed the presence of a Baker's cyst. I was referred to an orthopedist. After examining my knee, the orthopedist told me the cyst had been caused by arthrosis. According to him, nothing could be done other than to insert an artificial knee in three or four years, by which time my knee would have become totally unusable.

When I received this diagnosis in August 2007, I had been on Dr. Seignalet's diet for two months, and the pain I used to feel in my hands was history. Over the next months, the Baker's cyst disappeared, and the pain in my knees gradually reduced as long as I was mindful of my current capacities as I exercised on the treadmill. At that time, I used to go for slow walks, and in the fall of 2008, I noticed that I felt neither the itchy sensation nor the pain. I then decided to walk a little faster. Since the winter of 2008–09, I go downhill skiing without elastic knee braces, and I can even take on steep slopes without feeling that my knees will give up if I attempt one more descent, as had previously been the case. The improvement in my knees and back joints took place so gradually that it took me quite a while to fully realize the extent of my relief. While it is nearly impossible to forget sharp pain, a state of well-being does not readily draw our attention, especially if it is attained gradually, and more so in a situation in which pain is intermittent.

4. ARTHRITIS/ARTHROSIS IN MY HANDS

At the beginning of 2004, I started experiencing piercing intermittent pain in the metacarpophalangeal joints, which link the bones in the hand called metacarpi to the bones in the fingers called phalanxes. This pain quickly became acute, and after a few months, I consulted a doctor. Because he did not observe any redness or swelling in the joints of my hands, he told me everything was okay.

The condition continued to evolve between 2004 and 2005, and acute episodes became frequent. At first, Tylenol would generally make the pain bearable. Quite rapidly, however, the pain became worse, and at the same time, I began to suffer serious insomnia. In November 2006, as I recovered from a cold that had lasted far too long, all the metacarpophalangeal joints on both hands began to hurt really badly. (The general weakening of my body and of my immune system may have caused the progression of the arthritis.) The pain then spread to the other two joints of the ring finger and of the little fingers, as well as those in the thumb. Simply pressing down on these joints would cause unbearable pain. Soon, I was totally unable to bend the two joints on my left thumb, while the right thumb could only bend to about a 50 percent radius. As for both ring fingers, they would bend to a maximum of only 90 percent, even if I put pressure on them. My little fingers suffered a major loss of their flexibility and bounced back like springs when I tried to bend them. In fact, I could no longer close my hands; I could no longer use them normally and felt virtually continuous and intense pain in the metacarpophalangeal joints. My joints had become so weak and sensitive that I was no longer able to open even a bottle of water. I had to use tricks to avoid handshakes, which had become real torture. Tylenol no longer relieved the pain. I tried various balms that are supposedly very effective against pain, but all in vain.

During my yearly physical checkup, my family doctor referred me to a rheumatologist. The only option I had was to consult with an internist. This physician prescribed Celebrex (100 mg), to be taken twice a day, because neither Tylenol nor aspirin could relieve my chronic pain. Celebrex provoked headaches that increased in intensity as the days went by, but my chronic pain did not subside in any noticeable way. What I eventually learned regarding the side effects and mode of action of Celebrex reinforced my decision to avoid this medication.[1] Despite all my efforts to acquire a better understanding of arthritis/arthrosis through reference books, recent scientific articles, the Internet, information provided by professional associations, nutritional counsel, etc., I could find no solution to my chronic pain. I also consulted with therapists in alternative medicine who had helped me find relief when I had suffered pain in my back, neck and knee. Unfortunately, osteopathic, acupuncture and kinesitherapy treatments managed to reduce the chronic pain in my hands for only a few hours.

PUTTING THE HYPOTOXIC
DIET TO THE TEST

1. HOW I DISCOVERED DR. SEIGNALET'S WORK

My discovery of Dr. Seignalet's work was no coincidence. I was
very worried by the arthritis/arthrosis I had suffered from for
three years because conventional medicine brought me no relief.
Since I would accept neither the pain nor the gradual loss of my
physical abilities, I was bent on examining all possible solutions to
my problem. Conscious of the role diet plays in the onset of many
diseases, I asked myself if my eating habits could be at the root of
my condition. Among other things, I suspected that some of the
foods that I ate might act as cofactors in the development of chronic
inflammatory disease. In medicine, a cofactor is an element that
cannot, on its own, cause a disease, but which, in association with
a genetic predisposition, can trigger a disease. For example, to
trigger rheumatoid arthritis, one has to be genetically predisposed to it; that is, one must have a particular genetic abnormality
that favors its emergence. A genetic predisposition in itself cannot
cause rheumatoid arthritis, though. There must be another factor:

for instance, an environmental factor. And in a broad sense, food is part of the environment.

But even if I supposed that some foods could be cofactors in the onset of arthritis, I had absolutely no way of determining which ones were causing my arthritis. I knew that I was intolerant to eggs and nuts if I ate them more than once a week, but eliminating them completely from my diet did not alleviate my chronic pain. I kept mostly to the principles of a good diet, but I believed that it was possible that certain foods—generally considered healthy—could, in some cases, be harmful due to genetic predispositions or personal sensitivities. Also, it was very difficult to determine the amount of time needed to evaluate the benefits of *not* eating a particular food. To find information on foods that are potential cofactors in arthritis, I did a great deal of research using scientific search engines as well as Google, but I did not find any pertinent answers.

At the beginning of June 2007, exasperated by my unbearable pain, I attempted a new search on the Internet. This time, I was determined to find relevant information on foods that were possible cofactors in chronic inflammatory disease. After a few hours of research, I came across Dr. Jean Seignalet's[1] website. This doctor had been both a clinician and a researcher, and he had specialized in rheumatology, immunology and nutritherapy. To me, all that was very positive. In addition, his diet was based on the elimination of two food groups that I consumed daily in abundance. I immediately got a copy of his book, *L'Alimentation ou la troisième médecine*, so that I could try his hypotoxic diet (also named the ancestral diet).[2]

2. THE HYPOTOXIC DIET: THERAPEUTIC EFFECTS ON THE ARTHRITIS/ARTHROSIS IN MY HANDS

On June 10, 2007, I started the hypotoxic diet, which prescribed the elimination of all animal dairy products and derivatives, all cereals (wheat, barley, corn, rye, etc.,) and more particularly, whole grains and their flour, with the exception of buckwheat flour and rice flour. Sesame grains were also allowed. I increasingly preferred to cook vegetables by steaming, and as much as possible, I ate them raw. I was far from believing that this diet would really help me. But instead of doing nothing at all, I thought it would be better to try it for three months, the shortest amount of time Dr. Seignalet recommended to evaluate its efficiency.

Since I ate butter, milk, cheese, yogurt and whole-wheat bread every day, the abrupt elimination of these foods was a real sacrifice. However, the desire to ease my pain and to escape, even a bit, from the hell of pain was so strong that I did not hesitate—I deprived myself completely of these cherished foods. To my great surprise— and despite my skepticism—just ten days after I started the diet, I no longer felt pain in my hands. Only when I applied pressure to my finger joints, and particularly to the metacarpophalangeal joints, did I feel pain. This sensitivity started to ease after three months on the diet, mainly in those finger joints that had been least affected by arthritis. As the sensitivity to pressure eased, without my having done any exercises, I slowly started to regain the capacity to use my hands. Three months after I began the diet, I could manipulate my thumbs and bend them far enough to touch the little finger. After six months, I was able to bend my thumbs at both phalanges. After twelve months, I was able to fold my ring fingers and my little fingers, although the third phalanges could not yet bend over my hand. After sixteen months, I was able to fold the extremities of my fingers (the third phalanges) on the inside of my hand and I no longer felt any pain when applying pressure to the metacarpophalangeal joints of those fingers that had been most affected (thumbs, ring fingers and little fingers).

This recovery of the normal use of my hands was unexpected. While Dr. Seignalet is very affirmative about the efficiency of his diet in eliminating chronic pain and in slowing disease progression, he is extremely prudent in his statements on the recovery of lost functions. He makes one point very clear: his nutritional diet does not heal the disease; however, it puts an end to its symptoms and stops its development, as long as one sticks with the diet. Therefore, to maintain its benefits, this diet must be followed for the rest of an individual's life, for it does not result in a cure but rather a remission of disease.

According to Seignalet, chronic inflammation generally appears after years of consuming foods that are harmful to certain genetically sensitive individuals. For example, we know that celiac disease occurs in genetically predisposed individuals, who, in about 95 percent of cases, are carriers of genetic molecules called HLA-DQ2 and/or -DQ8. HLA molecules usually allow the body's defense system to discriminate between the self and the nonself, but in this situation, HLA-DQ2 and -DQ8 send a wrong message to the T lymphocytes. When activated by a component of gluten called α-gliadin, the T lymphocytes will direct their attacks not only against this peptide but also against a protein component of the small intestine's mucosa. A gluten-free diet will stop the activation of T cells by the α-gliadin, and therefore the attacks against the small intestine's mucosa will also stop, and the individual's celiac disease will go into remission.

Depending on different genetic abnormalities, some people will suffer from rheumatoid arthritis, and others will suffer from symptoms of fibromyalgia or from any other inflammatory disease. But even if one cannot change one's genetic heritage (that is, a predisposition to contract a particular disease), one can eliminate the cofactors from one's diet (such as α-gliadin) that contribute to triggering the disease. Dr. Seignalet's greatest achievement was that he highlighted two families of cofactors that are responsible for triggering a number of diseases classified under the term *arthritis* (and that also trigger a number of other diseases).

Although the hypotoxic diet needs to be followed throughout a lifetime, once the diet has unclogged one's system, some people may occasionally deviate from it without major problems, as long as doing so does not become a habit. Naturally, it's a matter of personal sensitivities, and each individual must pay attention to his or her personal reactions. However, any deviations must be only occasional. For example, one of Dr. Seignalet's patients gained remission from her severe rheumatoid arthritis by following the hypotoxic diet but saw her condition deteriorate because she introduced the daily consumption of one small whole-wheat cookie. Luckily, by abandoning this habit, she was able to stop the reactivation of her disease.

3. THE HYPOTOXIC DIET: GENERAL EFFECTS ON MY ARTHRITIS

I have no doubts about the fact that in ten days, Dr. Seignalet's hypotoxic diet completely eliminated the arthritis/arthrosis pain in my hands. Also, the diet enabled me to completely regain the normal use of my hands in sixteen months. In fact, the only trace left is the slight loss of flexibility in the joints of my ring finger and the little finger of my right hand, which manifests in my not being able to completely close this hand at these two fingers. It is also clear to me that it is thanks to the diet that my knee joints regained their flexibility and their strength. As for my cervical spine (neck), the situation is more than encouraging, as I have not had any pain there at all since the end of 2008. At the level of the lumbar vertebrae, I consider my situation 90 percent improved. The pain shows up only occasionally, if I go overboard. Except on very rare occasions, the pain is quite mild compared to what I used to bear before. I am particularly thankful for the fact that after really prolonged periods of sitting, I am now able to stand up from my seat, to straighten up and go, without any difficulty.

4. METHODOLOGICAL CLARIFICATIONS ABOUT THIS BOOK

All scientific articles cited in this book were obtained exclusively from databases like PubMed, MEDLINE and Google Scholar. None of the scientific articles cited by Seignalet are mentioned in this work, as they were incorporated into his texts. The reader can read the summaries of the articles cited in this book on the website of the United States National Institutes of Health (NIH), National Library of Medicine: www.ncbi.nlm.nih.gov/sites/entrez. The names of the articles' authors can be entered into the site's search box with or without the date of publication (for example, citing the authors' names as follows: Visser J, Rozing J), the complete title of the article or the title and the periodical/volume number (for example, *Eur J Nutr,* 41, 2002, 132–137). It is also possible to consult complete articles in university medical libraries or to buy them online.

The primary objective of this book is to build awareness of Dr. Seignalet's teachings and to make them accessible to all. To accomplish this goal, I have lightened and simplified Dr. Seignalet's principles and theories. On advice from my main critics, I added illustrations to help with understanding complex notions.

I did an exhaustive literature review of recent scientific material to verify that Dr. Seignalet's theories are in harmony with more up-to-date results from scientific research in nutrition and chronic inflammatory disease. As readers will notice, not only do the numerous scientific articles cited confirm the validity of Dr. Seignalet's theories, but they also provide new data that corroborate it. My literature review was also meant to persuade health professionals of the importance of a targeted diet in treating people suffering from chronic inflammatory diseases. Numerous scientific works have shown that certain foods recommended by nutritionists are particularly harmful to certain groups of people. In the light of new data showing the importance of a targeted diet in maintaining good health, it is not surprising that modifying one's diet can result in a remission of many chronic inflammatory diseases (which have so far been considered untreatable) and also bring about the disappearance of their accompanying pain.

Works like those of Dr. Richard Béliveau[3] have shown that a targeted diet can prevent and treat certain cancers. The world of medicine needs to consider different means, other than medication, to prevent and treat chronic diseases and eliminate their associated pain.

3

CLINICAL TESTING AND RESULTS

1. WHO WAS DR. JEAN SEIGNALET?

Jean Seignalet (1936–2003) was an intern at the Montpellier Hospital in France and was also deputy head of clinics, senior lecturer and practitioner at Montpellier's Faculty of Medicine. He was a renowned specialist in immunology and led the human leukocyte antigen (HLA) laboratory in Montpellier from 1969 to 1999. He also had a degree in gastroenterology and another in hematology.

From 1959 to 1968, Dr. Seignalet practiced medicine, sometimes as a specialist and sometimes as a generalist. From 1968 to 1983, he concentrated on research, particularly in the fields of immunology and genetics, but continued some clinical activities. He was a pioneer in kidney grafting. In 1983, while still pursuing research, he returned to practicing general medicine. According to him, this dual culture provided him with a solid base in many branches of medicine, including general medicine, and enabled him to develop a vision of nutritherapy in relation to chronic inflammatory diseases. Before he focused on nutritherapy, Dr. Seignalet was very much appreciated as a scientist by his colleagues. He published more than 230 articles, with 78 of these appearing in international journals with review boards. He was troubled by conventional medicine's inability to truly help those suffering from chronic inflammatory disease, and from 1983 on, he dedicated himself to studying the role food plays in this type of disease. He conducted an exhaustive review of the body of scientific literature on the topics that were likely to be linked to physiology, chronic diseases and nutrition, and he started laying the foundation of the diet referred to as "hypotoxic" or "ancestral." His greatest achievement was that he successfully combined knowledge and different theories in a way that enabled him to develop a diet capable of halting many chronic inflammatory diseases.

Scientific principles, influences and Seignalet's development of the hypotoxic diet

Seignalet was mostly influenced by the works and theories of visionary doctors who not only were very creative but also had a great deal of empathy for their patients:

1) Dr. Edward Bach (1886–1936), originally from Great Britain, underlined the major role the intestines play in preserving health and the relationship between chronic disease and certain bacteria from intestinal flora.

2) Dr. Paul Carton (1875–1947), of French origin, constructed a theory of deposition and elimination processes as a cause of chronic diseases.

3) Dr. Catherine Kousmine (1904–1992), from Russia, did her medical studies in Switzerland. She exposed the dangers of industrialized preparation of food and the role that it plays in the development of chronic degenerative diseases. She also highlighted the existence of an intestinal porosity as well as the importance of the pH level in urine, which is an indicator of the acid-base balance of the body-fluid buffer system.

4) Dr. Jacques Fradin (1954–), of French origin, founded the Institute of Environmental Medicine, Paris (1987), and discovered that factors such as a shortage of omega-3 fatty acids, high-temperature cooking, consumption of dairy products, cooked cereals and lipophilic toxins were likely at the root of the steep rise in degenerative pathologies.

5) Dr. Guy-Claude Burger (1934–), a Swiss-born physicist, put forward (among other researchers) a theory that human enzymes were unadapted by nature to certain foods that we now consume. Dr. Burger defended the principle of eating foods raw.

Early tests

In 1985, Dr. Seignalet began testing the hypotoxic diet on volunteer patients suffering from serious chronic inflammatory diseases that conventional medicine could not control. The diet soon achieved results far beyond his expectations, not only in terms of the number of remissions attained but also the number of diseases for which remissions were attained. Patients came from all over France to consult with him. Dr. Seignalet scrupulously documented his results and attempted to publish them in the journals that usually accepted his works. However, his articles on the hypotoxic diet were systematically turned down. They no longer qualified for publication in scientific journals under the pretext that the testing they documented had not been carried out using the "double-blind" methods that are customary in the evaluation of medication.

The double-blind method requires that there be no possible distortion in the interpretation of results; therefore, no one—neither the patient nor the health professional administering the medication—must know who among the patients is receiving the active molecule or the inactive molecule (that is, the placebo). Double-blind studies make it possible to evaluate with the utmost efficiency medications or molecules that can be introduced into a pill, such as vitamins.

But the double-blind method is not suitable for the analysis of a complete diet. How is it possible to completely control what the patient eats? How is it possible that neither the health professional nor the patient knows the diet the patient is following? Also, for ethical reasons, Dr. Seignalet was opposed to confining any patients in his studies to a control group and thereby excluding them from the benefits of his diet.

The placebo effect

Some people might think that Dr. Seignalet's results could have been due to the placebo effect. A close look at the numerous studies carried out on the placebo effect clearly indicates that it is very variable and generally limited to subjective evaluations of pain.[1] Also, meta-analyses of the placebo effect have provided a new perspective on the real value of placebos. A systematic review by A. Hróbjartsson and P. Gøtzsche of thirty-two clinical trials in a study including 3,795 patients, during which patients were randomly given either a placebo or no treatment, did not show any significant clinical effects of the placebo. In the second part of this review, a meta-analysis was also carried out involving eighty-two clinical trials and continuous follow-up of 4,730 patients. Placebos had some benefits, but these benefits diminished when the number of patients involved was much higher.[2] The difference between placebo and no treatment at all was very significant when the issue being measured was subjective in nature (for example, self-reported pain, which is difficult to quantify) and was insignificant when the issue was objective (for example, the quantitative analysis of the presence of a certain substance in the blood). In an analysis by Vase, Riley and Price of thirty-seven studies (a group of twenty-three studies using only placebo as a control condition, and another fourteen studies investigating placebo analgesic mechanisms), it was found that placebos had minimal benefits, corresponding to a reduction in pain intensity of 6.5 millimeters on a scale of 100 millimeters. (That is, researchers show patients a scale in millimeters calibrated from 0 mm to 100 mm and ask the patients to rate the intensity of their pain on this scale.) The authors concluded that there was little evidence that, in general, placebos have a significant clinical effect.[3] In another meta-analysis based on fifty-two new studies on the placebo effect, Hróbjartsson and Gøtzsche[4] once again concluded that they did not find any evidence of a significant, generalized clinical effect due to placebos. They did, however, agree that there could be a very small effect on certain patients, especially as far as pain is concerned. Other recent, well-controlled experimental studies targeting the duration of the placebo effect on pain reduction strongly suggest that the placebo effect is very short-lived.[5] All these studies show that no placebo can produce a success rate of about 80 percent, like the rates obtained by Dr. Seignalet in his treatment of ninety-one chronic inflammatory diseases. In addition, many of Dr. Seignalet's cases achieved a remission from their disease that lasted for many years.

Epidemiological studies

The most common scientific method used to evaluate the effects of a diet is epidemiological study: a comparison of two individuals with different eating habits. Results are analyzed to identify any major tendencies. (This method was used to show that the virgin-olive-oil—based Mediterranean diet significantly reduced the risk of cardiovascular diseases.[6]) Multiple factors are involved in epidemiological studies, so in order for them to be reliable, they must be carried out over many years and must include a large number of people. Of course, doing so requires large sums of money—amounts that Dr. Seignalet did not have at his disposal. Significantly, as he excluded all cereals (except rice and buckwheat) and all animal dairy products from his diet, he could hardly get any research grants from government agencies, due to the economic importance of dairy products and bread in the French food industry.

In general, the medical establishment opposes using nutrition as a treatment for diseases. Dr. Caldwell B. Esselstyn, a renowned American surgeon who showed in a twelve-year study that a change in diet was more efficient than surgery in treating heart diseases,[7] affirms that "the simple fact that many patients can have a say in their own health is a challenge for some doctors. They find it difficult to intellectually accept that patients can take care of themselves with more drive and security, and that this can last long."[8] According to Esselstyn, eliminating toxic foods is crucial in the fight to improve the health of Americans. To make this happen, the bodies that establish public dietary guidelines must base their decisions on science. However, the United States Department of Agriculture is subject to intense lobbying by industry, which compromises its capacity to be fair and objective.[9]

Testimonial There are many testimonials on the Internet by people who successfully followed Dr. Seignalet's hypotoxic or ancestral diet. Dr. Seignalet's official website also presents many testimonials, as does the Passeport-Santé website.[10] In this book, I cite Julie's testimony in its entirety because it was of particular interest to me: it gives us an idea of Dr. Seignalet's personality. This testimonial was found in 2007 as a result of a Google search.

> Posted on 21-10-2003 at 15:01 by Julie
> I have been reading the exchanges here for weeks, hesitating to intervene.
>
> I heard about the death of Dr. Seignalet in mid-July and I was overcome with deep pain and consternation, and a deep feeling of injustice.
>
> I am one of those who got healed in a spectacular way by his hypotoxic diet and I shall eternally be grateful to him. As is the case with all other diseases the diet treats, it is only a permanent remission and the diet needs to be followed for life. Normally,

auto-immune thyroiditis constantly gets worse (destruction of the thyroids) and patients usually have to increasingly take hormones for life. Mine was stopped because it was identified at the early stage, in the inflammatory phase, but before any destruction of the thyroid had taken place. For one year now, I do not take any medication, and my hormone levels are not only back to normal, but are even better than they were before the onset of the disease. I do not exclude the chances of a reoccurrence, but I do not believe there would be one. I notice that my endocrinologist does not agree with me on the effects of the diet even though he has no other explanations to give me...conventional medicine is not ready to accept these types of methods that are too simple, too inexpensive, too general, too exact and that question the enormous pharmaceutical and food industry. Apparently there are also some people who become very aggressive as a result of this. It could be because this method makes them responsible for themselves. They would rather swallow pills or be followed up...But why would they (patients and physicians) not just TRY? repeated Dr. Seignalet.

His death did not shake my determination, nor my confidence in the efficiency of his diet, not one bit—neither for me nor for any of the few people I know, who have either been healed or who have improved remarkably because of his diet. Statistics on his success in a good number of diseases considered incurable (does not mean terminal) by conventional medicine are also impressive. I knew Dr. Seignalet as his patient and I can affirm that this modest man, who walked you to the door with a warm handshake in place of requesting payment, was anything but proud. No charisma, no imposition from this man who almost irritatingly implicitly delivered the message: I have explained it to you, now the ball is in your courts. His immunological, clinical and statistical approach was very serious. Now each one should pick and choose from his ideas that have been clearly proposed with a "maybe a little too general" hypothesis. It would be an error to confuse the medical aspects with the ideology. Dr. Seignalet has left us information that we hope physicians would continued to use and expand on.

2. THE HYPOTOXIC DIET: THEORETICAL BASIS AND PRACTICAL OBSERVATIONS

Dr. Seignalet noticed that chronic inflammatory diseases (often referred to as "degenerative diseases") were becoming more and more common, and that conventional medicine was either incapable or nearly incapable of treating them. According to Seignalet, lack of knowledge about the pathogenesis of many diseases explains why medicine currently focuses on treating the symptoms instead of the causes of disease, which poses a problem for physicians. He asked himself, "How is it that with all the major progress that has been made in the different sciences, we still are unable to explain the mechanism of so many diseases?" He also affirmed that medicine's increasing complexity had led most clinicians and researchers to narrow areas of specialization. As a result, they master only a few facets of a pathological state. This partial vision keeps them from seeing the general picture.

By contrast, Dr. Seignalet was schooled in different branches of medicine in addition to his activities as a clinician and researcher, which gave him a solid basis from which to carry out his research in nutritherapy. Also, as a clinician, he dedicated many hours each week to reading medical articles on different aspects of medicine such as rheumatology, gastroenterology, endocrinology, psychiatry, dermatology, ophthalmology, pulmonology, cancerology and dietetics. As a researcher, he oriented his reading towards the following areas: immunology, genetics, anthropology, bacteriology, molecular biology, physiology and the biology of aging, with particular attention to cellular physiology and the small intestine, especially its walls and bacterial flora. With the foundation of his combined experience, readings and reflections, he elaborated a hypothesis on the pathogenesis of more than ninety diseases considered partially or totally inexplicable.

According to his hypothesis, often the primary cause of chronic inflammatory disease is the modern diet. He distinguished three varieties of mechanisms likely to cause chronic inflammatory diseases:

1) *Autoimmune* pathology; that is, diseases that develop when certain cells and molecules of an individual's immune system attack his or her own cells and tissues.
2) *Deposition* pathology, which is triggered by the progressive accumulation in certain tissues of wastes or toxic molecules from large bacterial molecules or from insufficiently digested food. (These molecules can cross the walls of a small intestine if it has become very permeable.)
3) *Elimination* pathology, which occurs when molecules that cannot be degraded by human enzymes become too numerous to be efficiently eliminated by the different eliminatory organs (mainly represented by the kidneys, the liver, the skin, mucosa, the lungs and the intestines).

All the diseases whose progression has been halted by the Seignalet method result from one or two of these conditions.

Clinical testing

In 1985, Dr. Seignalet carried out the first tests of the hypotoxic diet and obtained his first recorded success with a patient suffering from rheumatoid arthritis. In 1988, after he observed during three years the effect of the diet on different patients suffering from this disease, he drafted his first theory of the pathogenesis of rheumatoid arthritis, and in 1990, he revised it, taking most autoimmune diseases into consideration. Thereafter, he set out to verify his theories by treating patients suffering from fibromyalgia, arthrosis, type 2 (non-insulin-dependent) diabetes, psoriasis, Crohn's disease and asthma, among others.

In 1994, he extended his deposition hypothesis to include other malignant diseases, having found that his theory could be applied to about 66 percent of cancer cases. Whenever he thought that his diet could combat a certain disease, he enlisted any volunteers ready to try his method, especially those with unbearable, treatment-resistant pain. After eighteen years of clinical application of his hypotoxic diet and eighteen years of obtaining numerous extremely positive results—documented in successive editions of his book, *L'Alimentation ou la troisième médecine*—Dr. Seignalet showed in his book's fifth edition, published in 2004, one year after his death, that the hypotoxic diet had a major therapeutic effect on many diseases. In this last edition, he describes his experience as he followed 2,500 patients, demonstrating the effect of his diet on ninety-one chronic diseases, with a success rate of about 80 percent. He also reported that his diet did not work for twenty-four other diseases. In this edition of *L'Alimentation ou la troisième médecine,* Seignalet revised some of his theories. His conclusions were more solid, as he now had a much broader perspective, given the large number of patients who had applied his nutritional principles for at least five years. In addition, a close examination of the documented causes of failure in some diseases can help to partly or totally enlighten us on the mechanisms of these diseases.

The main findings of his studies highlight the multifactorial nature of the ninety-one diseases that responded positively to his method: they depend on both genetic factors and environmental cofactors. A disease can be identified as multifactorial by carrying out studies on identical twins. For example, a study of rheumatoid arthritis on a group of identical twins can show that when one twin suffers from this disease, there is a 15 percent risk that the other twin could suffer from this disease as well—compared to a 1 percent risk for the general population. Therefore, even though there is a hereditary factor involved, one or more cofactors must be present for the disease to manifest. The cofactor could be linked to the environment, as in the case of a particular food, for example; in which case, we refer to a multifactorial disease.

3. DISEASES THAT RESPONDED POSITIVELY TO THE HYPOTOXIC DIET

Dr. Seignalet tested his hypotoxic diet on 115 diseases, 91 of which responded positively. The effects of the hypotoxic diet on 43 of these diseases were observed in 2,390 patients, for an average of 55 patients per disease. The effects of the diet on 43 other diseases that responded positively were observed in a total of 188 patients only, for an average of about 4 patients per disease. For this reason, only the results obtained with the 43 diseases that affected a reasonable number of patients are presented in the tables below. Table 1 presents the list of autoimmune diseases; table 2, the diseases Dr. Seignalet classified as diseases of deposits (Dr. Seignalet lists Alzheimer's, myocardial infarction, cancer and gallstones in this category because his hypotoxic diet had a marked preventive effect on these diseases); table 3 covers diseases he referred to as elimination-related diseases.

TABLE 1: Autoimmune diseases

DISEASE	NUMBER OF PATIENTS	COMPLETE REMISSION	REMISSION ≥ 90%	REMISSION ≥ 50%	FAILURE RATE (%)	SUCCESS RATE (%)
Systemic lupus erythematosus	20	10	6	3	1	95
Rheumatoid arthritis	297	127	100	18	52	82
Polymyalgia	17	12	4	0	1	94
Psoriatic arthritis	39	15	10	11	3	92
Inflammatory rheumatism	15	12	0	2	1	93
Sjögren's syndrome	86	15	11	48	12	86
Scleroderma	14	0	14	0	0	100
Multiple sclerosis	42	13	20	8	1	98
Ankylosing spondylitis	122	76	40	0	6	95
Acute anterior uveitis or iridocyclitis	14	10	2	0	2	86

TABLE 2: Deposition diseases

DISEASE	NUMBER OF PATIENTS	COMPLETE REMISSION	≥ 90% REMISSION	≥ 50% REMISSION	FAILURE RATE (%)	SUCCESS RATE (%)
Tonsillitis	15	14	0	1	0	100
Osteoarthritis	118	47	52	12	7	94
Tension headache	15	11	3	0	1	93
Endogenous depression	30	25	0	5	0	100
Diabetes mellitus type 2	25	20	0	5	0	100
Dyspepsia	63	62	0	1	0	100
Unexplained tiredness	10	5	0	3	2	80
Fibromyalgia	80	58	10	4	8	90
Parkinson's disease	11	0	7	3	1	91
Migraine	57	41	12	0	4	93
Osteoporosis	20	progression arrested in 14 cases				70
Spasmophilia	52	46	2	1	3	94
Overweight	100	30	21	21	28	72
Hypoglycemia	16	13	0	1	2	87
Hypercholesterolemia	70	68 patients experienced at least a 35% drop in cholesterol levels				98
Tendinitis	17	13	2	0	2	88

* Prevention of Alzheimer's disease, myocardial infarction and cancer as demonstrated by statistical studies (see p. 38)

TABLE 3: Elimination diseases

DISEASE	NUMBER OF PATIENTS	COMPLETE REMISSION	≥ 90% REMISSION	≥ 50% REMISSION	FAILURE RATE (%)	SUCCESS RATE (%)
Cystic acne	42	40	2	0	0	100
Canker sore*	14**	10	4	1		100
Asthma	85	80	0	3	2	98
Chronic bronchitis	42	39	0	3	0	100
Colitis	237	233	0	0	4	98
Allergic conjunctivitis	30	26	1	2	1	97
Atopic dermatitis	43	36	4	0	3	93
Gastritis	19	18	0	1	0	100
Recurrent ENT infections	100	80	0	0	20	80
Crohn's disease	72	62	2	7	1	99
Angioedema	27	22	2	2	1	96
Psoriasis	72	45	7	8	12	83
Chronic rhinitis	63	58	0	3	2	97
Hay fever	75	71	0	2	2	97
Chronic sinusitis	50	38	0	8	4	92
Gastric reflux disease	16	6	5	0	5	69
Hives	34	29	5	0	0	100

* Superficial mouth ulcer
** This figure corresponds to the one published in Dr. Seignalet's book. It is possible that it should be 15.

Complex diseases classified separately

• Behcet's disease: 12 patients, 100 percent success rate

Diseases (number: 43) that responded positively to the hypotoxic diet on a limited number of patients (between one and nine):

- Still's disease
- chronic juvenile polyarticular arthritis
- chronic juvenile oligoarticular arthritis
- palindromic rheumatism
- dermatomyositis
- polymyositis
- mixed connective tissue disease
- cutaneous lupus
- fasciitis "Shulman's syndrome"
- chronic relapsing polychondritis
- Graves' disease
- Hashimoto's thyroiditis (when treated before the destruction of glandular thyroid cells)
- celiac disease
- Peyronie's disease
- autoimmune hepatitis
- primary biliary cirrhosis
- primary sclerosing cholangitis
- pemphigus
- Guillain-Barré syndrome
- peripheral neuropathy
- Wegener's granulomatosis
- polyarteritis nodosa
- autoimmune Addison's disease
- gout
- chondrocalcinosis
- autism
- dystonia
- arthritis of the lower limbs
- medullary aplasia
- glaucoma
- idiopathic pulmonary fibrosis
- microscopic colitis
- ulcerative colitis
- urticarial vasculitis
- pruritus
- sinonasal polyps
- histiocytosis
- cutaneous mastocytosis
- IGA nephropathy (blockage of progression)
- Palmoplantar pustulosis presenting with chest pain
- SAPHO (synovitis, acne, pustulosis, hyperostosis and osteitis syndrome)

The hypotoxic diet and Alzheimer's disease, myocardial infarction and cancer

Seignalet carried out statistical studies evaluating the effects of his hypotoxic diet on Alzheimer's disease, myocardial infarction and cancer. He proceeded by documenting, over a long period, the number of cases of Alzheimer's, myocardial infarction and cancer present in 1,200 of his patients treated with nutritherapy. He compared this group to a control group involving about the same number of people of the same origin and age group, but who had never been on the hypotoxic diet. His studies revealed the preventive effects of the hypotoxic diet: while he observed no cases of Alzheimer's disease among his group of patients, there were 30 in the control group; he observed 5 cases of myocardial infarction in his group of patients, compared to 28 in the control group; and lastly, he observed 3 cases of cancer among his patients compared to 30 cases in the control group.

4. DISEASES THAT RESPONDED NEGATIVELY TO THE HYPOTOXIC DIET

- amyloidosis
- Addison-Biermer anemia
- juvenile diabetes type 1
- contact dermatitis
- monoclonal gammopathy
- chronic lymphocytic leukemia
- Churg-Strauss disease
- erythremia
- melanomas
- myasthenia gravis
- narcolepsy
- alopecia areata
- idiopathic thrombocytopenic purpura
- ulcerative colitis
- sarcoma
- sarcoidosis
- multiple chemical sensitivity
- chronic fatigue syndrome
- myelodysplastic syndrome
- thrombocythemia
- benign tumors
- Hashimoto's thyroiditis (unless the diet is begun at the very onset of the disease)
- vitiligo

4

KEY ELEMENTS OF DR. SEIGNALET'S DIET

It is well known that the different components of the human body are continually renewed and that the substances needed for this process are drawn from food. Cells also draw the energy that they require for proper functioning from food. As a result, our choice of foods has great influence on the proper functioning of our bodies. If we consume too many foods that our system is unable to properly digest and that our eliminatory and excretory organs (the kidneys, liver, lungs, intestines, skin and mucosal membranes) are unable to handle, wastes accumulate in the body and hamper normal metabolism. Dr. Seignalet showed that diseases that responded well to his nutritional method were caused both by a genetic susceptibility and by environmental factors. Among environmental factors are certain foods that act as cofactors and that trigger diseases that are partially genetic in origin. Our modern diet causes an imbalance in the small intestine due to the accumulation of too many improperly digested food molecules that promote the growth of pathogenic bacteria to the detriment of saprophytic (good) bacteria.

Ninety percent of diseases that have the common trait of a mysterious mechanism and resistance to conventional treatments are caused by this imbalance. Unlike the hunter-gatherer prehistoric human's food, the modern diet relies on the consumption of cereals, large quantities of milk products (especially in North America), reared meats and cooked foods. Of course, prehistoric humans ate meat, but they ate raw meat from wild animals, which means that the meat had a lot less fat than the meat we consume today.

In the middle of the last century, the dawn of industrialized agriculture and cattle rearing brought about an even greater change in diet. Obviously, industrialization and globalization greatly modified farming methods and ways of feeding animals, which affected the quality of foods (see chapter 6, section 5).[1]

Finally, as we've increased our consumption of industrially processed foods, refined sugar, salt, fats and chemical substances since the 1960s, overweight, obesity and chronic diseases affect an increasing percentage of the population.

According to Dr. Seignalet, the primary cause of these malfunctions is the inability of human digestive enzymes and mucins (glycoproteins contained in intestinal mucus) to adapt to the modern diet. This inability promotes the accumulation of wastes and harmful bacteria in the small intestine, provoking an increased permeability that allows the transfer of harmful molecules from bacteria and food into the blood and tissues. These changes, depending on genetic susceptibility, may induce deposit pathologies or autoimmune and elimination diseases. It is therefore essential for us to know which foods suit our systems and which foods we must avoid.

1. ENZYMES
The role of enzymes in the digestion of food

Enzymes are proteins produced by cells. The role of enzymes is to activate biochemical reactions in living beings. Food provides most of the molecules on which enzymes act or that influence enzyme activity. Enzymes accelerate the speed of a reaction, act in very small quantities and remain intact at the end of reactions. Enzymes are very specialized molecules, and so there are many of them. Each enzyme recognizes a specific site on a substrate (that is, the molecules on which the enzymes act) and provokes a specific type of reaction. Enzymes play a primary role in Dr. Seignalet's hypothesis regarding the diseases his diet successfully treats. According to Seignalet, enzymes are helpful in explaining both the mechanisms of these diseases and their prevention and treatment.

Enzymes: Their mode of action

To be able to act, an enzyme must be placed in specific conditions. Complementarity between an enzyme and its substrate must be very precise. An enzyme can be compared to a key and the substrate to a lock. Once the enzyme and substrate associate, two factors encourage enzyme activity: 1) temperatures generally close to 37°C (99°F); and 2) an acidity level corresponding to a pH lower than 7 or an alkalinity level corresponding to a pH higher than 7. The optimal pH level varies with the enzyme involved. For example, while the pepsin enzyme, whose role is the degradation of proteins in the stomach, requires a pH level of 2 to 4, which is very acidic, trypsin, which plays the same role in the small intestine, requires a pH level of 8 to 9, which is very alkaline.

Because enzymes are very strong molecules that can damage the tissues of the host organism if they are not properly controlled, many mechanisms are involved in their inhibition or activation. A great majority of enzymes decompose substrates like food in the small intestine. Humans possess an arsenal of enzymes, but the efficiency of many enzymes will vary between individuals according to personal heredity. An individual in whom certain essential enzymes do not function as well as they should would be more prone to autoimmune diseases and deposit pathologies than another in whom these essential enzymes function properly.

The enemies of enzymes

The principal enemies of enzymes are excess free radicals,* pesticides, various medications (including antibiotics), tobacco, air pollutants, water and soil. However, according to Seignalet, the worst enemies of digestive enzymes are molecules from modern foods that these enzymes are unable to digest. As these foods accumulate in the small intestine, their molecules encourage the multiplication of patho-genic bacteria; consequently, the integrity of the small intestine's walls is compromised, increasing their permeability.

Consequences of enzymatic dysfunction

When enzymes can't reduce food molecules to a sufficiently small size, putrefaction happens in the intestines, causing a dispropor-tional increase in harmful bacteria, which in the long run, affects the integrity of the small intestine's walls. The dysfunction of diges-tive enzymes is one of the main causes of the onset of autoimmune disease and deposit pathologies. Deposit pathologies (particularly glycotoxin deposit) could affect both the extracellular and intra-cellular environment. Glycotoxin deposition can more or less completely block certain enzymatic cascades; that is, a series of bio-chemical reactions mediated by enzymes in a precise way. Taking this fact into consideration, it becomes easier to identify foods that must be excluded to prevent or heal numerous diseases—diseases that have so far been deemed difficult to treat or incurable.

---

*   Free radical: Any atom or molecule that has a single unpaired electron in an outer shell. For most biological structures, free radical damage is closely associated with oxidative damage.

2. THE IMPORTANCE OF SMALL-INTESTINE INTEGRITY IN MAINTAINING GOOD HEALTH
Characteristics of the small intestine

The small intestine is a key organ. It ensures that foods are digested, while its epithelial mucosa serves as a barrier between the internal milieu of the human body and the nutritive and other elements from the environment. The small intestine ensures the absorption of water and nutrients. The integrity of the intestinal barrier is crucial for normal physiological functions and for the prevention of sickness. In certain individuals, the barrier does not play its role properly and lets through too many macromolecules that have not been sufficiently degraded by digestive enzymes. These substances are sometimes harmful, and in cases in which there are hereditary predispositions, their accumulation can encourage the onset of many diseases.

The small intestine is about 5 to 6 meters (16 to 20 feet) long, and its mucosa consists of an epithelium made of only one layer (¼₀ millimeter) of cells called enterocytes. When a cross-section of the small intestine is examined, numerous folds (appendix 1a) that carry intestinal villi (appendix 1b) can be seen. The functional surface of the villi of a small intestine is more than 100 square meters. Each villus contains an arteriole, a capillary network, a small vein and lymphatic vessels (appendix 1c). Cells of the intestinal epithelium (the enterocytes) are welded to each other with different types of junctions. Junctions referred to as tight junctions play a particularly important role because these links between the epithelial cells of the mucosa serve as barriers to insufficiently digested molecules, which are too big and are harmful[2] (appendix 1d).

In healthy individuals, the unmodified tight junctions of a mature intestine play a key role as they are the principal barrier against macromolecules. Different elements like cytokines, hormones and other molecules play the role of messengers and regulate the function of junctions between the enterocytes, ensuring the passage of small molecules into the inner milieu.

Other cell types in the intestinal epithelium

There are different types of cells in the epithelial walls of the small intestine: M cells, which could play a primary role in specific immunity in relation to antigens located inside the intestine, and goblet cells, which specialize in the secretion of mucus (appendix 1c). Mucus helps maintain the integrity of the intestinal mucosa and aids in the scarification of its wounds. It is composed of a protective gel that is insoluble in water and a viscous layer made up of glycoproteins that are soluble in water, including mucins. This insoluble gel constitutes a physical barrier between enterocytes and microorganisms and other harmful elements. A third kind of cell, Paneth cells, would secrete, in a retaliation response to pathogens, a large array of antimicrobial peptides against bacteria, fungi, protozoans and viruses.[3] Finally, intraepithelial lymphocytes are located at the base of the epithelial layer of the intestine. These lymphocytes are exposed to a great variety of microbial and nutrient antigens, and they protect the host against invasion by microorganisms that penetrate the gastrointestinal tract.

Main functions of the small intestines

The small intestine takes part in the digestion of food by breaking down, through the action of digestive enzymes, large complex molecules into small simple molecules. Polysaccharides are broken down into simple sugars, lipids are broken into simple fats, and proteins into small peptides and amino acids. The small intestine ensures the selective absorption of broken-down substances through the villi. The products of digestion can go through the intestinal barrier in two ways. Most absorbed proteins (= 90%) go

through the intestinal barrier and directly penetrate the enterocytes with the help of microvilli (appendix 1d). These proteins are
then degraded by enzymes into lysosomes, which digest them into
molecules too small to provoke an immune response.[4] Only the
remaining little peptides and amino acids can pass between the
enterocytes by the intermediary of tight junctions (appendix 1d),
which are precisely regulated to help prevent immune reactions.[5]
Direct passage through the enterocytes happens with the help of an
active transport that requires a bout of energy, while molecules go
through the tight junctions between the enterocytes by a passive
transport. The intestinal barrier's integrity can be compromised
by abnormalities in the tight junctions located between the epithelial cells. When altered, tight junctions (appendix 1d) cannot
effectively block the passage of large bacterial or nutrient molecules,
and these molecules then cross the intestinal mucosa and can cause
the onset of autoimmune or allergic disease.[6]

Finally, products of digestion in the form of average chains—
that is, only partly digested—are drained by blood and pass through
the liver. Products of digestion of lipids are drained by the lymph.
Food substances and other substances that are not completely
digested are called chyle. Chyle goes through the small intestine
into the colon. The contraction of smooth muscles, referred to as
peristalsis, propels the ball of food through the intestines, with the
process facilitated by the presence of mucus. Peristalsis is similar to
a unidirectional wave, provoking successive narrowing that pushes
food down into the extremities of the digestive tube.

Bacterial flora of the small intestine

The human digestive tract contains about 10^{14} bacteria (that is, hundreds of billions), approximately ten times the total number of cells
in the body. These microorganisms normally stay confined in the
intestines. There are up to about 10^{11} microorganisms per gram of

content, while there are between ten and some hundreds of organisms per gram of substances contained in the first part of the small intestine. This number increases in the last part of the small intestine that precedes the large intestine.[7] This microflora is essential for the normal development and functioning of the digestive tract and the immune system, since it ensures the maturation of the intestinal immune system.[8] Bacteria in the colon are anaerobic in nature, meaning that they do not need oxygen and that in 99 percent of cases, their activity depends on fermentation. In the first two parts of the small intestine—the duodenum and the jejunum—there are bacteria that are aerobic in nature; that is, they require oxygen to grow. Anaerobic bacteria are predominant in the ileum, the last part of the small intestine.

A total of about 400 to 500 species of bacteria live together in the intestines. Some of the bacteria are there only temporarily, while others live there permanently. A diet rich in meats encourages development of a flora of putrefaction, while a vegetarian diet promotes a flora of maceration. In its normal state, the bacterial flora that colonizes the intestines is a saprophytic flora, meaning that the bacteria live in harmony with the human body—in symbiosis with it. These bacteria complete the digestion of certain foods, break down bile pigments, participate in the fabrication of vitamin K, slow the development of yeasts and fungi, and liberate polyamines (molecules whose amino groups have more than one function), which are nutritive for enterocytes when available in physiological doses. Sometimes the bacterial flora become pathogenic and encourage the onset of disease. In such cases, one or more dangerous bacteria overdevelop and provoke diseases either by secreting toxins or by crossing the epithelium of the intestinal mucosal membrane. Bacteria that die in the small intestine decompose into peptides and lipopolysaccharides (molecules made out of sugar molecules and lipids), as well as other, more or less dangerous substances, especially when they cross the epithelium of a mucosal membrane that has become too permeable.

We have seen that tight junctions located between the endothelial cells of the small intestine regulate the transport of nutritive molecules towards the internal environment of the body by preventing the migration of large food and bacterial molecules, and the movement of microorganisms across the intestinal membrane.[9] However, this selective permeability can be directly altered by bacteria or indirectly altered by cytokines produced by the immune response of the host.[10] Obviously, an overgrowth of bacteria in the small intestine can facilitate the transfer of these bacteria or their antigenic components through the intestinal barrier, which can harm one's health.

Defenses of the small intestine

The small intestine can be compared to a very thin but immense filter, for the cells of the mucosal membrane, referred to as enterocytes, are set out in only one layer. They are, however, the only barrier that separates our internal environment from certain harmful agents from the environment present in the small intestine: parasites, bacteria, viruses, foods.

The defense mechanism of the small intestine consists of nonimmune first-line defenses such as gastric acidity (which has bactericidal characteristics), digestive enzymes and bile, intestinal motricity, saprophytic bacteria that oppose the multiplication of pathogenic germs, intestinal secretions of antimicrobial peptides and mucus capable of neutralizing pathogens.

The immune cells disseminated in intestinal mucosa are white blood cells named leukocytes. Leukocytes responsible for the specific immune response come from a lymphoid bone-marrow cell. These leukocytes are made up of B lymphocytes, plasmocytes gotten from B lymphocytes that secrete antibodies that can recognize an antigen in a very precise manner, and long-life memory cells (appendix 2). The second group of leukocytes responsible for

specific immunity is made up of T lymphocytes, which when activated by an antigen specific to them, differentiate themselves into
1) auxiliary T cells that secrete cytokines; 2) killer T cells, referred
to as cytotoxic cells; and 3) memory T cells (appendix 3). Another
lineage of cells related to lymphocytes consists of NK (natural killer)
cells, but these cells do not possess any antigenic specificity. B and
T lymphocytes are mostly concentrated in lymphoid tissues like
lymphatic ganglions. Leukocytes responsible for the innate or nonspecific immune response can also be found there. These leukocytes
come from a myeloid stem cell of bone marrow and consist of
monocytes/macrophages, mast cells, dendritic cells and the polymorphonuclear group of leukocytes that include neutrophils,
eosinophils and basophils (appendixes 4 and 5).

The need for immune tolerance

The mucosal membrane of the small intestine constitutes a
protective—but imperfect—barrier against foreign antigens. In
a healthy, average adult, macromolecules such as lipopolysaccharides, peptides and even proteins can generally cross the intestinal
wall in relatively small quantities with no serious adverse effects
(which is what we mean when we speak of immune tolerance). In
small children, however, this phenomenon can more frequently
cause an immune response due to the greater permeability of the
immature intestine. Therefore, there is generally immune tolerance towards foreign antigens when the quantity of macromolecules
crossing the small intestine is very small or negligible.

Hyper-permeability of the small intestine

Since the 1980s, we've known that even in healthy individuals, the
imperviousness of the small intestine is imperfect and that small peptides can cross the intestinal barrier as easily as amino acids. Even

proteins cross the mucosal membrane in small, but non-negligible quantities. We talk about hyper-permeability of the small intestine as a pathological condition when large quantities of food proteins cross the intestinal mucosa. Thus, intolerance to cow's milk and gluten can be observed in a number of adults. Migraines caused by milk, wheat and eggs are healed by eliminating those foods from one's diet. According to Seignalet, an increase in the small intestine's permeability was proven in most of his patients who were suffering from chronic inflammatory disease.

Causes of hyper-permeability of the small intestine

Seignalet indicated that the tract that cuts across the enterocytes in the small intestine is solid and rarely disturbed; meanwhile, the weakest link in the intestinal mucosa is the tight junctions that join the enterocytes to each other. It has been demonstrated that a fast-growing number of diseases involve alterations in intestinal permeability—alterations that are related to changes in tight-junction competence (appendix 1d).[11] Foods from the modern diet to which our digestive enzymes are ill adapted can help to create a predisposition to small-intestine hyper-permeability. Anti-inflammatory medications—the most well known of which include salicylates (like aspirin) and ibuprofen (like Advil)—corticosteroids and certain antibiotics may also damage the walls of the small intestine. Antibiotics are particularly harmful when used over a long period: in certain individuals, they can cause a real dilapidation of the small intestine by deeply modifying its bacterial flora and altering the cells of the intestinal mucosa. The effect of these different factors is the excessive multiplication of pathogenic bacteria that destroy the cells of the intestinal mucosa and can cause serious lesions with inflammation.

Researchers recently showed that other hormonal factors like cytokines can also weaken the small intestine by altering the lipid composition of its cellular membranes, and in particular, those of its tight junctions. In fact, cytokines are messenger molecules that manifest as small peptides produced by cells of the organism— generally, cells of the immune system, and usually in response to the presence of pathogenic microorganisms. Certain cytokines have the ability to remarkably increase the permeability of the small intestine's mucosal membrane by loosening the tight junctions between enterocytes, which allows large, insufficiently digested molecules to cross the interior of the intestines into the blood and lymphatic circulation and into the interstitial fluid in which the cells bathe. Other enemies of the small intestine are excess free radicals, pesticides, certain pollutants, radiotherapy and chemotherapy, as well as the medications listed above.

Genetic characteristics and the development of small-intestine hyper-permeability

To maintain its physical and physiological integrity, an organism must set up strategies that enable it to avoid being engulfed by cells, molecules or foreign organisms. Evolution has endowed our bodies with a system of recognition that makes it apt to differentiate between the "self" and the "nonself" by the intermediary of glycoproteins called HLA (human leukocyte antigen), which are incorporated into the surface of most of its cells. HLA molecules are part of the large gene family of major histocompatibility complex (MHC): genes that are specialized in the recognition of "self" and "nonself." The term HLA applies solely to molecules of human MHC. MHC genes encode for class I and class II HLA molecules. When an HLA molecule associates with a "nonself" antigenic substance (or one considered thus), this association is highlighted by a recognition and signaling system that commands all the specific immune cells to fight the invader as a "nonself." HLA-I molecules have the task of reporting the presence of any endogenous antigens (such as tumor antigens) coming from a transformed cell or from a cell affected by virus parasites or intracellular bacteria. These antigens are treated like "nonself" antigens since they differ from the antigens of this normal cell. However, these foreign antigens are obviously from an endogenous source since they were produced in the very interior of the HLA-I carrier cells (appendix 6). On the other hand, HLA-II molecules have the task of reporting the presence of any antigenic substances and germs that have entered the body through a wound or a highly permeable or wounded intestine. These antigenic substances come from outside the body and are therefore of exogenous origin and represent substances of the "nonself" group (appendix 7). Apart from a few exceptions, such as mature red blood cells, all the cells of an individual carry class I HLA molecules. Class II HLA molecules, however, are generally present only on APC cells whose function is to present antigens to T lymphocytes that carry specific receptors capable of recognizing particular antigens. Cells that are able to play the role of antigen-presenting cells (APC) are dendritic cells, macrophages and B lymphocytes. HLA molecules are defined by the genetic baggage inherited from each of our parents. Each child, therefore, in part differs from or is similar to each of his or her parents with regard to their HLA molecules; and consequently, individuals more or less differ from each other, except for identical twins.

One of the principal factors that cause excessive permeability of the small intestine is the genetic fragility towards certain antigens. As such, class II HLA molecules like HLA-DQ2 and HLA-DQ8, when associated with certain antigens from the environment, can deliver incorrect messages that can, in turn, lead the immune system to err. Celiac disease is a good example of genetic fragility towards a factor in the environment: in this case, the α-gliadin, a peptide derived from the digestion of gluten and found in many cereals (appendix 8). In such instances, immune antigen-presenting cells (APC) that express HLA-DQ2 or -DQ8 molecules can activate T lymphocytes in an abnormal way. Consequently, the activated T lymphocytes will attack not only the gliadin molecules but also one type of protein present in the intestinal mucosa. This situation leads to the onset of a chronic autoimmune and inflammatory disease named celiac disease. Bear in mind, though, that the HLA-DQ2 or -DQ8 molecule cannot trigger the immune disease on its own. The disease will occur only if the sensitive HLA is associated with one or more environmental or random factors able to activate T-specific T lymphocytes that have the potential to trigger the disease.[12] Susceptibility to at least fifty diseases has thus been associated with specific HLA alleles in the presence of one or more triggering environmental factors.

Consequences of the hyper-permeability of the small intestine

As a consequence of the small intestine's hyper-permeability, excessive quantities of antigenic molecules from insufficiently digested food, along with pieces of bacteria and sometimes even whole bacteria, can cross the walls of the small intestine (appendix 9). The tight junctions of the intestinal epithelium, once they've been modified by microbial infections or by an overstimulation of the immune system, allow these substances to penetrate general circulation and to lodge in different tissues and parts of the body. Combined with certain genetic factors, these macromolecules can lead to the onset of chronic inflammatory diseases (appendixes 8 and 9).

3. DATA FROM RECENT MEDICAL RESEARCH CONFIRMING THE ROLE OF HYPER-PERMEABILITY OF THE SMALL INTESTINE IN THE ONSET OF CHRONIC DISEASES

Autoimmune diseases are of particular concern in the Western world. They affect 5 percent to 8 percent of the American population: between 14 million and 22 million individuals. In the United

States, they stand third among the most widespread diseases, after cancer and heart disease.[13] Improper functioning of the tight junctions of the intestinal epithelium seems to be the primary problem in many autoimmune and/or chronic inflammatory diseases.[14] There appears to be a direct relationship between the Western diet and the epidemiologic prevalence of autoimmune and/or chronic inflammatory diseases. The number of patients suffering from chronic inflammatory diseases like ulcerative colitis and Crohn's disease started increasing in Western Europe and North America amid the economic growth that followed the Second World War. Many epidemiologic studies on the Western lifestyle since 1990 have suggested that environmental factors such as mass-produced food and intestinal germs play a determinant role in the pathophysiology of inflammatory diseases of the intestine.[15]

Japan and intestinal inflammatory disease

In 2008, an analysis of epidemiologic data related to the Japanese population showed that the number of patients suffering from Crohn's disease and ulcerative colitis was increasing following the adoption of Western dietary practices about twenty years earlier.[16] Although in the 1970s Crohn's disease and ulcerative colitis were very rare among the Japanese, at the end of the 1980s, the number of Japanese suffering from ulcerative colitis was close to 20,000, and those suffering from Crohn's disease numbered about 5,000. In 2000, 60,000 people suffered from ulcerative colitis, and 20,000 from Crohn's disease. In 2006, the last year of the compilation, cases of ulcerative colitis numbered 90,000; and for Crohn's, they reached 25,000.[17] Such considerable changes in a short time and in a large number of individuals can only result from environmental factors, as genetic changes take place over very long periods.

An analysis of the epidemiological data in this study high-lighted the following points:

1) Westernized food could have affected the intestinal germs, which could have led to changes in the intestinal epithelium.
2) Intestinal germs could be responsible for the onset of inflammatory diseases of the intestines.
3) There seems to have been a latent period of about twenty years between the start of the Westernized diet and the manifestation of inflammatory diseases of the intestine.
4) The most remarkable changes to the Japanese diet were an increase in foods from animals and a reduction in the consumption of rice.
5) A strong incidence of Crohn's disease was observed between the second and the third decades of life, and for ulcerative colitis, between the third and fourth decades. It therefore takes approximately two to three decades for the symptoms of these diseases to manifest in humans.
6) Long-term exposure to the antigens in the intestines is necessary before the first clinical signs of these diseases appear.

This study shows that twenty years after the start of nutritional changes, the increase in daily consumption of meat and animal fats, of milk and milk products, as well as the concomitant reduction of rice consumption, is linked to a marked increase in the cases of ulcerative colitis and Crohn's disease in the Japanese. When the evolution curves of foods consumed by the Japanese from the 1950s are closely examined, the three most remarkable facts are the drop in the consumption of rice, which moved from about 350 grams per day to about 160 grams per day in 2002; the increase in the consumption of milk and milk products, which went from less than 10 grams per day to about 135 grams per day; and the increase in the consumption of meat, which went from less than 10 grams per day to close to 70 grams per day in 2002.[18]

The West and intestinal inflammatory disease

In Western countries, the majority of infectious diseases of the intestines are generally under control while food allergies and idiopathic inflammatory conditions (that is, diseases of unknown causes) have increased dramatically. In other words, these are inflammations without infection, a characteristic observed in chronic inflammatory diseases. The role of the microbial flora of the small intestine, including pathogenic and commensal microorganisms, in the maintenance of good health or in the onset of chronic disease has been recognized for some years now. Inflammatory diseases of the intestines in particular, such as Crohn's disease, ulcerative colitis and celiac disease, have been the object of many research projects. Regarding the onset of inflammatory phenomena that seriously damage the intestinal mucosal membrane and increase permeability of the intestinal epithelium, there is consensus on the role that bacterial flora plays.[19] If intestinal microbial flora can cause such damage in certain individuals, it is due in part to environmental factors like nutritional styles and also in part to genetic characteristics that affect immune-system function at the level of the intestines.

Examples of autoimmune diseases due to gluten intolerance

Gluten—and more precisely, a peptide called α-gliadin that is present in wheat, barley, rye and related cereals—acts as a triggering environmental agent of celiac disease. In individuals genetically predisposed to celiac disease, immune antigen-presenting cells (dendritic cells, macrophages, and B lymphocytes) carry on their surface genetic molecular markers called HLA-DQ2 or -DQ8. The presence of this genetic particularity, which plays a role in the recognition of self and nonself, provokes, as mentioned above, aberrations in the recognition of certain antigens (appendix 8). T lymphocytes then react by inducing an excessive secretion of pro-inflammatory cytokines. The action of these causes the tight junctions of the intestinal epithelium to release, which increases permeability of the intestinal mucosa. Molecules that should normally not cross the intestinal barrier can then make it through and provoke disease.[20] Very early in the development of celiac disease, the tight junctions are open[21] due to the disorganization of the proteins of which it is made, causing severe intestinal damage.[22] Perturbation of tight-junction proteins is directly caused by exposure to gliadin.[23] Much evidence suggests that an increase in intestinal permeability also plays a central role in the pathogenesis of other inflammatory diseases of the intestines. It has also been observed in a certain number of Crohn's patients that an increase in permeability of the intestinal epithelium occurred about one year before the clinical stage of the disease.[24] This finding indicates that excess intestinal permeability is an early event in the development of the disease.

Halting the autoimmune process

Initially, it was believed that once the autoimmune process was activated, it was irreversible.[25] A new theory suggests that the autoimmune process can be halted if the proper functioning of the intestinal barrier is restored after the elimination of the environmental factor or factors that interacted negatively with the genetic factors responsible for predisposition to autoimmune diseases.[26] The removal of gluten from the diet of individuals genetically susceptible to celiac disease brings a gradual repair of the intestinal mucosa and recovery of the normal function of the intestines. The effects of a gluten-free diet show that environmental factors are at least as important as genetic susceptibility[27] in the development of celiac disease.

Type 1 diabetes and intestinal flora

It is well established that the development of type 1 diabetes results from both a genetic susceptibility and environmental factors. Unlike type 2 diabetes, type 1 diabetes is insulin dependent: it is an autoimmune disease that destroys the insulin-secreting cells of the pancreas. A great deal of recent data suggest that genetic susceptibility to type 1 diabetes leads to the disease in the presence of the following environmental factors: an abnormal intestinal flora, a too-permeable intestinal mucosa and an alteration in the immunity of the intestinal mucosa.[28] The presence of commensal intestinal flora (normal flora that participates in the proper functioning of the intestines) in infancy is critical for normal physiological development, as well as proper development and stimulation of both the adaptive immune and innate immune systems.[29] Scientific studies on laboratory animals have shown that changes in microbial flora can lead to the onset of autoimmune diabetes and that taking probiotics can cause the secretion of anti-inflammatory cytokines that prevent the development of type 1 diabetes in NOD (nonobese diabetic)[30] mice.

Hyper-permeability of intestinal mucosa

Studies have shown that a person's tendency to develop type 1 diabetes or another autoimmune disease is usually linked to an abnormally permeable intestinal barrier,[31] which is due to the alteration of tight junctions located between the intestinal mucosa's epithelial cells.[32] The increased permeability of the intestinal mucosa leaves the intestinal immune system more exposed to foreign antigens,[33] which in turn encourages the development of type 1 diabetes.

Intestinal immunity

The third element that plays a key role in the development of type 1 diabetes is intestinal immunity. We know that 80 percent of immune cells reside within the intestinal wall. A well-balanced microbiome (intestinal flora) favors the development and the activation of a normal immune system. For example, the immune systems of children who are born by natural means and breast-fed are better able to protect them from autoimmune diseases and allergies.

Biopsies on children with type 1 diabetes show an abnormal activation in the system of cytokines in the lamina propria, the site where immune cells reside below the intestinal epithelium.[34] In individuals suffering from type 1 diabetes, there have been more reports of an aberrant response to food, which is shown in an increased immune response towards wheat and cow's milk, which can favor inflammation of the intestines.[35] This type of reaction is based on the same general principles described above for the abnormal immune response to α-gliadin in celiac disease. This phenomenon was not observed in biopsies on healthy children.[36] However, once the disease is established, a diet that excludes these substances does not modify the autoimmune response of patients suffering from type 1 diabetes.[37] Currently, it's suspected that enteroviruses (viruses that enter an organism through the gastro-intestinal system) could trigger intestinal immunity problems in patients suffering from type 1 diabetes. Therefore, enteroviruses, by modifying the secretion of cytokines, can cause an increase in the permeability of the small intestine, which could lead to an increased sensitivity towards food proteins.[38]

A pilot study of children genetically susceptible to type 1 diabetes, carried out over a mean observation period of 4.7 years, showed that it was possible to reduce autoimmune reactions against the cells of the pancreas (those that secrete insulin) by 50 percent when the children were nourished with a hydrolyzed casein-based formula (a milk protein decomposed into its different amino acids) for a minimum of six to eight months instead of with an ordinary cow's-milk[39]–based preparation. The study's authors believe that this dietary modification will normalize the composition of microbial intestinal flora, thereby diminishing intestinal permeability, and by this very fact, reduce the inflammatory response, since exposure to nutrient antigens would be delayed until the intestine matures sufficiently.

Fibromyalgia and intestinal flora

Fibromyalgia, a condition of hypersensitivity of the musculoskeletal system, eloquently shows the link between the overgrowth of bacteria in the small intestine and cells' hypersensitivity in general.[40] The intensity of pain caused by fibromyalgia correlates to the amount of bacterial overgrowth in the small intestine.[41] This disease is usually linked to an increase in intestinal permeability.[42] Intestinal hyper-permeability directly corresponds to the development of fibromyalgia, since the food or bacterial substances crossing an altered intestinal mucosa come into contact, in an abnormal manner, with the intestinal and extraintestinal immune system.[43] Later on, these substances can stimulate the immune system cells that cause systemic diseases like intestinal inflammatory diseases, allergies and arthritic diseases.[44] There should be a link between fibromyalgia and irritable bowel syndrome, given that between 30 percent and 70 percent of patients suffering from fibromyalgia also have symptoms of irritable bowels.[45] The role that intestinal germs play in fibromyalgia is suggested by two studies that showed that between 84 percent and 100 percent of patients suffering from fibromyalgia had tested positively for the production of hydrogen methane gas.[46] These observations suggest that an excessive increase in bacteria in the small intestine and an abnormal intestinal microbial flora can contribute to inducing a somatic or visceral hypersensitivity in patients who have been diagnosed with irritable bowel syndrome or fibromyalgia, or both.[47]

Rheumatoid arthritis and intestinal flora

Rheumatoid arthritis is an autoimmune disease in which the immune system attacks the joints. Inflammation starts at the envelope of the joint—the synovial membrane or synovium—and generally provokes pain, gradually leading to permanent lesions. The disease can affect the eyes, lungs and heart.

Studies analyzing the relationship between diet and rheumatoid arthritis are rare and often contradictory, which can be explained by the complexity of epidemiological studies.[48]

A 2007 research study confirmed the thesis that rheumatoid arthritis results from a reaction to food antigens and that the disease's process begins within the intestines.[49] This finding confirms earlier studies that showed that a meatless diet, without gluten or cereals and with no milk products, leads to improvement in the symptoms of rheumatoid arthritis patients.[50] Notably, a study carried out on 82,063 women between 1980 and 2002 eliminated red meat, chicken and fish as factors likely to trigger rheumatoid arthritis.[51] This study strongly suggests that it is the elimination of dairy products and gluten that improves the symptoms of rheumatoid arthritis patients—not the elimination of meat.

In the 2007 study mentioned above,[52] a group of patients suffering from active rheumatoid arthritis followed, for two weeks, an elementary diet (a diet that excluded proteins and was made up of only amino acids, mono-/disaccharides and triglycerides with added vitamins and traces of minerals). The control groups, made up of patients also suffering from active rheumatoid arthritis, were treated with 15 mg of prednisolone per day for two weeks. (Prednisolone is an anti-inflammatory medication administered for periods not exceeding two weeks[53] to patients suffering from

rheumatoid arthritis.) At the end of the study, all clinical parameters normally evaluated in rheumatoid arthritis patients had
improved for the two groups, except for swelling of the joints in
the elementary-diet group. Results show that the elementary diet is
as efficient as treatment with an anti-inflammatory drug like prednisolone in improving the clinical signs of rheumatoid arthritis.
This study supports the thesis that in individuals with a genetic
predisposition, rheumatoid arthritis results from a reaction with
food antigens, with the pathology originating in the intestines.[54]

A team of researchers led by Alan Ebringer has been trying for
many years to show that there is a link between the bacteria *Proteus
mirabilis* and rheumatoid arthritis.[55]

This link would be represented by similarities between protein
antigens that belong to both *Proteus mirabilis* and host-tissue antigens. As a consequence of these similarities, an immune response
directed at first against a microbial pathogen would be redirected
against certain host tissues. This phenomenon, known as molecular
mimicry, ties in with Dr. Seignalet's basic hypothesis that bacterial
infections are at the root of hyper-permeability of the small intestine and also that certain bacterial antigens cause autoimmune
reactions. However, *Proteus mirabilis* would not be the only microorganism that has similarities to host proteins.[56] As mentioned
above, genetic susceptibility to autoimmune reactions depends on
risk factors such as the presence of certain HLA molecules on the
surface of cells—molecules that somehow constitute a passport that
establishes the "self." We now know that individuals who carry the
HLA-DR14 antigen on their cells are likely to develop rheumatoid
arthritis. We also know that genetic predisposition alone is not
enough to cause the disease: there must also be an environmental
trigger. In this case, it is possible that a *Proteus mirabilis* infection
acts as a trigger by causing the formation of lymphocyte clones
(that had previously been sequestrated or prohibited because they
are related to the self), which then attack the collagen of the joints.[57]

Conclusion

Before the 1980s, conventional medicine hadn't realized the extent to which the human intestinal microflora played a determinant role both in disease and in maintaining good health. Our modern diet seems to disrupt homeostasis—the equilibrium of intestinal microflora—in a significant number of individuals who have genetic predispositions to inflammatory disease. Also, this phenomenon is becoming more and more common in older people. An individual's immune response might be disturbed due to the overgrowth of pathogen bacteria in his or her small intestine, especially if heredity has predisposed that individual to certain diseases. Thus, the clinical manifestations observed in many diseases can be explained by several factors: the modern diet, the host response and nutritional and bacterial antigens crossing through a too-permeable intestinal mucosa. To properly diagnose and effectively treat chronic inflammatory disease, it is essential to acknowledge the role played by the interaction between a host and its intestinal flora in the disease's development.

4. DR. SEIGNALET'S NUTRITIONAL THEORY AND THE CONTRAST BETWEEN ANCIENT DIETS AND THE MODERN DIET

The ancestral diet and the modern diet

The ancestral diet appeared during the Paleolithic Era, which corresponds to the period during which prehominids (biped primates who appeared approximately 25 million years ago) and then hominids (who appeared approximately 6 million years ago) evolved gradually into *Homo sapiens* (about 200,000 years ago). The diet of the hunter-gatherer, which developed during the Paleolithic Era, underwent radical transformations about 10,000 years ago, during the Neolithic Era.[58]

Hence, the dietary needs of humans were defined by natural selection for millions of years, during which time prehominid ancestors, then hominids and after that *Homo sapiens* consumed foods derived exclusively from wild animals and uncultivated vegetables.[59] This mode of feeding influenced the selection of current human genetic characteristics, such as the mass and form of the body, the capacity to move, the mastication apparatus, growth and developmental stages, the relative size of the brain, metabolic activities and particularly the specificity of digestive enzymes.[60] The passage to the Neolithic Era about 10,000 years ago corresponds to the period during which humans became sedentary. Three great changes resulted from this development: the domestication of cereals, principally wheat and barley; the breeding of goats and cows that produce milk; and the cooking of several foods. This period, which began with the Neolithic Era, represents less than 1 percent of the period that witnessed the evolutionary development of humankind. The changes that arose during the Neolithic Era have, in turn, resulted in the industrial production of food during the last two centuries.[61]

Given the slow pace of evolution, the changes tied to agriculture and industrialization came too fast for the human genome to adapt itself to them. Anthropological studies have established that present-day humans have the same genetic characteristics as Paleolithic generations, and that consequently, we are adapted to the nutritional mode of the period that preceded agriculture.[62] During the preagricultural period, humans were hunter-gatherer nomads who ate game, fish, fruits, vegetables, uncultivated plants and honey when possible. They consumed neither milk (except their mother's milk) nor dairy products, nor oils, salts, transformed foods or refined sugars. Compared to the present-day Western diet, food during the Paleolithic Era provided much more soluble and insoluble fiber, as well as two to ten times more micronutrients. In fact, cereal grains began to interact with the human genome only about 10,000 years ago, and except for humans, no free-living primates consume this type of food. Since the advent of agriculture, cereals such as wheat, rice and corn provide humans with 40 percent to 90 percent of their energy needs, contrary to what happened during the period preceding the development of agriculture.[63]

The industrialization of food

The twentieth century witnessed the development of the food industry, which ushered in changes in oil processing, livestock feeding, plant cultivation and animal rearing, as well as in culture, with the new methods often leading to deficiencies in vitamins and particularly in minerals.[64] Such radical changes in diet, taking place during such a short period in relation to the rate of human evolution, may explain the susceptibility to chronic disease that affects 50 percent to 65 percent of individuals aged fifty and above in most Western countries.[65] Diet-related chronic disease is extremely rare in hunter-gatherer peoples or in non-Westernized societies. One could counter that assertion by saying that the life expectancy of these populations is very inferior compared to that of industrialized countries, which would explain the differences observed. However, if we consider the years between 1950 and 1970 in Western countries, there is evidence that chronic inflammatory diseases such as type 2 diabetes, arthritis, cancers and heart diseases were much less common in people aged fifty and older than they presently are.

In summary, for millions of years, hominids and their descendants consumed non-transformed foods to which, during evolution, their enzymes and mucins had adapted. The modern diet, which dates back to the Neolithic Era, is rich in new molecules to which our enzymes and mucins are not necessarily well adapted. The situation got worse during the twentieth century, particularly since the 1980s, with the massive industrialization of food and the globalization of eating habits.

5. DOMESTICATED CEREALS: A FOOD ISSUE

According to references cited by Seignalet, cereals are vegetable species whose grains, either whole or reduced to flour, serve as food for humans and domestic animals. Plants considered to be cereals include wheat, barley, rye, oats, buckwheat, rice, millet, sorghum, corn and other related cereals. Most cereals are grasses, with buckwheats being among the exceptions.

Cereals contain 10 percent protein on average, little fats, lots of carbohydrates, mineral salts and vitamins. Hunter-gatherers already consumed wild carbohydrate grains during prehistoric times, but only in small quantities.[66] Currently, cereals make up two-thirds of the calories and half of the proteins absorbed by humans. The modern-day food pyramid based on grains is contrary to the feeding experience that corresponds to hominid evolution.

Changes in the structure of cereals

Cereals have undergone numerous modifications since the beginning of agriculture, and these changes are due to several causes: a) an initial selection from a population of wild grasses to retain only the forms suitable for cultivation; b) a selection that conserved, for future planting, only grains from the best ears and the biggest grains, which often resulted from genetic mutations (meaning that consequently their proteins could differ from those of the original grains); c) hybridization; and d) transplantation into a new environment, which implied a selection of the most adapted variants.

Modifications in wheat, rice and maize according to a review of the literature by Seignalet

About 10,000 years ago, the ancestor of wheat had a diploid AA genome with seven pairs of chromosomes. Hybridizations, mutations and recombinations led to hard wheat, which comes from a tetraploid cereal with 14 pairs of chromosomes. Hard wheat is used in making pastes and semolina. Kamut wheat, often said to be ancestral, is also transformed, as it has 14 pairs of chromosomes. Soft wheat has 21 pairs of chromosomes and is used in making bread, pizzas, croissants, cakes, cookies and wheat flour. Barley and rye have 7 pairs of chromosomes and are diploid; they would have had the same ancestors as wheat. Wheat is very close to barley, a little less so to rye and even less to oats. It is very distant from rice, maize and African cereals. Bread combines starch grains and proteins, some of which form a network called gluten during kneading. Rice has 12 pairs of chromosomes. Rice is different from the other cereals in that despite manipulations of it by farmers, it tends to return to its initial wild state. Modern rice is therefore more or less identical to prehistoric rice. Maize descends from teosinte, from which it differs by five major and several minor mutations. Wild maize does not exist anymore.

The harmful effects of cereals

Data cited by Dr. Seignalet indicate that wheat, and to a lesser extent, maize, have been implicated in several diseases: rheumatoid arthritis, multiple sclerosis, celiac disease, dermatitis herpetiformis, certain migraines, type 1 diabetes, schizophrenia and Crohn's disease.

Seignalet believed that the danger of cereals resides in the structure of certain proteins in wheat, maize and related cereals. These proteins would have undergone profound mutations during prehistoric times that, Seignalet affirmed, the enzymes and mucins of some humans were not well adapted to. He put forward the hypothesis that cereal proteins became harmful after cooking due to the transformations they undergo in the process. This hypothesis was tied to the fact that all cereal products are cooked or prepared by techniques requiring high temperatures. Seignalet asserted that rice proteins, even once altered by cooking, were much better tolerated.

Recent studies confirming the harmful effects of cereals

Seignalet's hypothesis on the harmful effects of cereals resulting from their transformation by treatment with high temperatures is now confirmed. Scientific results demonstrating the plausibility of this hypothesis are explained in detail in chapter 4, section 7. Several health problems related to the consumption of cereals have been uncovered following the discovery in 2003 of receptors for toxic products arising from high-temperature cooking of cereals. To begin with, wheat is one of the eight most allergenic foods that provoke more than 90 percent of allergic responses.[67] These allergies are associated with several wheat proteins, the most important being gluten.[68] However, intolerance phenomena, which unlike allergies do not necessarily involve the presence of antibodies specific to certain cereals, seem much more widespread than allergies. Thus, celiac disease (chronic inflammation of the intestine) affects 1 percent of the Western population,[69] while dermatitis herpetiformis would have an incidence rate somewhere between 0.2 percent and 0.5 percent.[70] Gluten acts as a cofactor in celiac disease, which affects genetically predisposed individuals: the predisposition concerns the HLA-DQ2 and HLA-DQ8 antigens in about 95 percent of patients, and the HLA-DQ8 antigen in about 6 percent of them.[71] Celiac disease therefore results from an autoimmune response triggered by gluten in certain genetically predisposed individuals.[72]

Autoimmune diseases such as rheumatoid arthritis occur more frequently in patients suffering from celiac disease and their families.[73] Also, associations between wheat, celiac disease and schizophrenia have been established.[74] Other associations between gluten sensitivity and neurological symptoms, despite the absence of damage to the intestinal mucosa, have been observed,[75] as has been the case with sporadic ataxia.[76] In addition, gluten sensitivity has been associated with eczema,[77] irritable bowel syndrome,[78] migraines,[79] acute psychosis[80] and other neurological diseases.[81] A relationship with autism has also been reported.[82] Some physicians recommend a gluten-free and dairy-free diet for children suffering from autism.[83]

A number of research studies suggest that gluten primarily affects the nervous system[84] in people who are genetically sensitive to gluten, which would explain why small quantities of gluten can cause serious pathological reactions, as well as a variety of symptoms. It is estimated that at least one out of ten people are affected by gluten.[85] In many cases, the disease is silent at the intestinal level and is not diagnosed. Therefore, to preserve the health of the whole community, it is crucial to properly understand the gluten syndrome.[86]

Gluten, in addition to several cereal proteins, is likely to trigger chronic inflammatory conditions that cause numerous diseases.[87]

6. THE PROBLEM WITH ANIMAL MILKS
The harmful effects of dairy products

For several million years, the ancestors of man and *homo sapiens* did not consume any other milk but maternal milk. Domestication of milk-producing species began about 10,000 years ago, and the consumption of animal milk and its derivatives would have begun during this period. The selection of milk-producing cows is relatively recent, and it is particularly from the mid-twentieth century that cow's milk and its derivatives began to occupy a prominent place in the nutrition of adults and children, particularly in America.

However, Seignalet affirmed that the regular consumption of milk products can have adverse health effects, including the development of chronic inflammatory diseases.

Breast milk and cow's milk

According to several authors, human milk is the only food really adapted for the needs of a newborn and a young child. When we compare a woman's milk with cow's milk, we see important differences in the development of an infant compared to that of a young calf. Thus, cow's milk contains 32 grams per liter (g/l) proteins, compared to 9 g/l for a woman's milk. Furthermore, casein represents 80 percent of the total protein in cow's milk, compared to 17 percent for a woman's milk—probably because the growth of a calf is much faster than the growth of infants, with calves doubling their birth weight in 36 days, compared to 105–126 days for infants.[88]

Cow's milk proteins and human diseases

Recent studies tend to demonstrate that the A1 variant of beta-casein, a protein, is particularly abundant in the milk of Holstein cows and other predominant races in our livestock. This variant could play a role in the development of human diseases.[89] Epidemiological studies conducted in New Zealand suggest that the consumption of A1 beta-casein is associated with a higher national mortality rate related to cardiovascular diseases. (The caseins are the most important proteins in cow's milk, where they account for 80 percent of proteins. Caseins play an important role in the toxicity of cow's milk. More articles cited demonstrate the differences between the casein found in cow's milk and breast milk and link it with cardiovascular disease.)[90] Another notable difference between human milk and cow's milk is the predominant presence in human whey of the protein alpha-lactalbumin, while in cow's milk the predominant protein is beta-lactoglobulin, which is absent from human milk.[91]

Development of the human brain and breastfeeding

Another major difference is that the carbohydrates and complex lipids found in human milk favor the much more complex development of the brains of infants, which develop more slowly than those of calves. This long maturation is related to the intellectual faculties of humans. A meta-analysis based on eleven controlled studies shows that human milk, in comparison to cow's milk formulas, is associated with a 3.2-point rise in children's intelligence quotients. This difference has been observed at age six months and has been maintained up till age fifteen, the oldest age considered in the study. In regard to cognitive development, the longer the period of breastfeeding, the greater the difference between the two methods of milk feeding.[92]

Protective effects of breastfeeding

Numerous studies have shown that breastfeeding protects against several pathologies. From a review of the literature covering the period between 1966 and 2001, we conclude that breastfeeding protects against atopic diseases or allergies. Other research suggests that breastfeeding guards against asthma, type 1 diabetes, Crohn's disease and ulcerative colitis.[93]

According to Seignalet, the fact that cow's milk contains three times more calcium and iron than breast milk is not without consequence. These minerals are poorly absorbed by the intestinal mucosa of an infant, which paradoxically sometimes leads to a deficiency in iron and calcium, while the infant who is breastfed suffers no such deficiency. Seignalet points out that the growth factors found in cow's milk are meant to enable the calf put on more than 100 kg (220 lb) in one year, which is unsuitable for a human being.

Recent research confirming the existence of relationship between milk products and chronic diseases

New data from recent research studies strongly support the hypothesis that animal milk favors the onset of chronic diseases in humans. According to Professor B.C. Melnik,[94] consumption of animal milk proteins is an environmental factor that helps to trigger most of the chronic diseases found in Western societies. Organizations dedicated to the promotion of healthy nutrition strongly recommend the consumption of milk and milk products, but it seems as if we have failed to consider the negative long- and short-term effects of these products on health. The particularly negative effects of milk products are largely due to the changes in hormonal equilibrium between insulin, the growth hormone, and IGF-1 (insulin-like hormone growth factor 1), the structure of which resembles that of insulin.[95] These changes lead to an increase in blood insulin and, consequently, a constant increase in the serum levels of the IGF-1 hormone as well as the development of type 2 diabetes and other chronic diseases in genetically predisposed individuals.

IGF-1 hormone and cancer

The IGF-1 hormone is a powerful mitogen (an activator of cell multiplication) that when linked to its receptor in various tissues induces cellular proliferation and inhibits apoptosis.[96] (Apoptosis is programmed cell death—cell suicide controlled by a signal.) In abnormal and/or cancerous cells, it is a particularly beneficial activity. Because the IGF-1 hormone can prevent suicide in abnormal cells, it has the characteristics of a tumor activator.[97] Different studies have demonstrated that there is a correlation between high serum IGF-1 levels and an increase in the incidence of colorectal cancer, as well as breast, ovarian, uterine, prostate and lung cancers.[98] Long-term studies carried out in Scandinavia involving 25,892 Norwegians clearly showed that daily consumption of more than 750 milliliters of milk yielded a relative risk of 2.91 of developing breast cancer when compared to a relative risk of 1.0, which corresponds to a neutral result.[99] Curiously, this 2.91 relative risk is not publicized. Meanwhile, the Women's Health Initiative[100] study that found a 1.26 relative risk of developing breast cancer after taking hormone replacement enjoyed a lot of publicity in journals and among medical doctors. Many patients discontinued a treatment that had improved their quality of life following the publication of this study, whose protocol had noticeable weaknesses, as gynecologist Sylvie Demers reveals in her book *Hormones au féminin*.[101]

Milk products and increases in blood insulin levels

Cow's milk contains 4 to 50 nanograms of active IGF-1 per milliliter (ng/ml). High levels of IGF-1 are still detectable after the milk is pasteurized and homogenized. Human and bovine IGF-1 have the same amino-acid sequences, and consequently bovine IGF-1 binds to human receptors.[102] High consumption of milk in humans is associated with a 10 percent to 20 percent increase in levels of circulatory IGF-1 in adults and a 20 percent to 30 percent increase in children,[103] which probably explains why milk products have an insulin index (that is, the increase in the quantity of insulin in the blood following the ingestion of a carbohydrate) that is three to four times higher than their glycemic index[104] (that is, the increase in the quantity of sugar in the blood following ingestion of a carbohydrate). This is true for skimmed as well as whole milk, indicating that the fraction of milk proteins is what is responsible for the increase in blood insulin levels.[105] The fact that even the intake of skimmed milk has been associated with type 2 diabetes points in the same direction.[106] Except for cheese, which has an insulin index two times less than that of milk (a characteristic that has not yet been explained), all milk products, including yogurt, ice cream, cottage cheese and products made from fermented milk, have strong effects on insulinemia.[107] Milk products increase the level of IGF-1 more than any other protein food source, including meat. One consequence of hyper-insulinemia is the acquisition of insulin resistance, which can contribute to an excessive increase in the weight of a newborn and favor obesity and type 2 diabetes.[108] These observations are supported by clinical results that show high serum IGF-1 levels in obese children. At two months, children who are breastfed have a serum

IGF-1 level of 93.3 +- 23.6ng/ml, while those who are fed with a cow's milk formula show an IGF-1 level of 129 +- 39.8 ng/ml.[109]

Stimulation of insulin secretion and the development of chronic diseases

According to an article by Melnik[110] in an issue of *Medical Hypotheses* that addressed all facets of this problem, the consumption of cow's milk, because it induces a strong stimulation of insulin and IGF-1 and an increase in insulin resistance, is contrary to physiological principles of human nutrition developed during evolution. Advocating consumption of cow's milk to promote bone formation and mineralization is short-sighted and does not take into account well-documented facts demonstrating the role played by cow's milk proteins in the development of cardiovascular diseases, type 1 diabetes, obesity, neurodegenerative diseases, acne, and atopic and autoimmune diseases, including different forms of arthritis and certain cancers. High levels of IGF-1 would promote the development of these diseases, as high levels have an inhibitory effect on the mechanisms of apoptosis. It is no coincidence that these diseases most particularly affect Western countries, where the consumption of cow's milk and dairy products is strongly encouraged. These works corroborate Dr. Seignalet's hypotheses: he believed that the composition of cow's milk evolved to accelerate the growth of the calf and did not suit the slow development of the human being and, particularly, the human brain.

Correlation between the high consumption of milk in children and type 1 diabetes

Official recognition of the harmful effects of milk would cause enormous economic repercussions, just as was the case for a very long time with cigarettes. So the powerful argument of "controversy" is put forward instead. To feed the controversy, the dairy industry uses the fact that the inclusion of cheese in independent studies weakens the relationship between the consumption of cow milk proteins and the development of type 1 diabetes. This argument is contestable, for it has been demonstrated that unlike other dairy products, cheese does not lead to a marked increase in insulinemia and in the level of blood IGF-1.[111]

Meanwhile, certain correlations seem much more valid: the consumption of cow's milk in children up to age fourteen in twelve countries correlates almost perfectly with rates of type 1 diabetes. This relationship was demonstrated in an analysis published in 1991, which indicated that 94 percent of the incidence of this disease could be explained by a difference in the consumption of cow's milk, according to geographic variation.[112] In Finland, where there is enormous consumption of dairy products, type 1 diabetes occurs thirty-six times more frequently than in Japan, where there is little consumption of dairy products.[113] According to a study carried out between 1990 and 1999,[114] a diagram indicating the incidence of type 1 diabetes in children less than fourteen years old, in fifty-seven countries, clearly shows that countries with the highest consumption of dairy products also have the highest annual incidence rate: more than fifteen diagnosed cases per 100,000 inhabitants. Canada comes sixth, with more than twenty cases of type 1 diabetes diagnosed per 100,000 inhabitants each year, while Finland comes first, with about forty cases per 100,000 inhabitants per year.[115]

According to Melnik, we need to be particularly concerned about the consumption of cow's milk during pregnancy and during the postnatal period. These are crucial times in the development of children, and that development should only be stimulated by growth factors produced by their own species. Hormonal changes during the first months of uterine life and postnatal life can affect an individual's health as an adult, predisposing that individual to cancer, allergies and other chronic diseases. Epidemiological, biochemical and clinical studies, as well as circumstantial evidence, support the hypothesis that the consumption of cow's milk is a great danger to health and should be recognized as being at the origin of most chronic diseases in industrialized countries.[116]

Chronic disease and accelerated industrialization of milk production

Between 1925 and 1955, type 1 diabetes was rare in Western countries.[117] However, the incidence of type 1 diabetes had increased annually by about 2.8 percent since the 1960s, corresponding to an increase in the consumption of dairy products.[118] Roughly the same period has seen an increase in chronic disease in the West, coinciding with the accelerated industrialization of food.[119] To increase milk production, particular breeds of cows were selected, their diet was changed and in many cases, the animals were raised "above ground" (that is, kept locked in a barn). In 1955, a French cow produced 2,000 kilograms of milk per lactation and met its feeding needs with prairie grass and hay. Today, the Prim'Holstein cow, widespread in our herds, produces an average of 9,100 kilograms of milk per lactation and can even surpass 11,000 kilograms per lactation. To attain this immense productivity, milk cows, which are herbivores, are fed grains containing carbohydrates that are rich in starch and rapidly absorbed, including corn, barley and soybeans, generally conserved by ensilage, as well as molasses and dextrose. These foods induce an insulin resistance in cows, which could result in the development of diabetes if the cow were allowed to live long enough.[120]

A resistance to insulin, and, most often, diarrheas are observed in calves when they are intensively milk fed.[121] Dairy cows are also given hormones and antibiotics to respectively increase their productivity and fight diseases, including mastitis, a common inflammation of the udder in these extremely productive cows. Dairy cows are called "animal machines" and are compared to "mechanical engines" as if they were cars.[122] Just how illogical our modifications of these herbivores' feeding habits has become was demonstrated by mad cow disease in the 1990s. This disease, properly called bovine spongiform encephalopathy, stemmed from bovine contamination through the consumption of bones and meat flours contaminated with nervous tissues of sick animals.

It is unrealistic to think that major dietary modifications in cows will not affect their milk and, therefore, dairy products. Is it merely coincidental that since the 1960s, the rates of type 1 diabetes and other chronic diseases have increased with the industrialization of food production, particularly milk production? One must also consider the fact that milk is sterilized at high temperatures. The harmful effects of treating foods with high temperatures will be discussed later in this chapter.

Dairy products and osteoporosis

Osteoporosis is a major health issue in the West. It is a disease that causes a weakening of the bones and an increased risk of fracture by reducing bone density and changing the micro-architecture of bone tissues. It has multiple causes such as genetic factors, hormone deficiency—mainly estrogen and parathormone—dietary habits, lifestyle and lack of physical exercise. This multiplicity is the reason why, even though calcium is an essential component of the skeleton, the development of a healthy skeleton is too complex to be limited to a mere intake of calcium and vitamin D. It's now evident that taking the appropriate quantities of calcium and vitamin D cannot efficiently protect one from bone loss, especially in old age.[123] Regular physical exercise is an excellent way to protect one's health as a whole, and starting from menopause, it is an excellent way to ensure bone strength.[124]

Because multiple factors are involved in the development of osteoporosis, it is difficult to discern the different interactions among these factors and to find a means of fighting the disease. However, presenting dairy products as a cure for osteoporosis because dairy products are rich in calcium and proteins is not justified. Many scientific studies have shown that despite an increase in the consumption of dairy products, the incidence of osteoporosis has noticeably increased in the last two or three decades. Osteoporosis affects about 25 percent of menopausal women in North America. In fact, one out of two women and one out of five men, aged fifty and over, will suffer a fracture due to osteoporosis at some point during the remainder of their lives.[125] Osteoporosis leads to a great number of fractures and contributes to the increase in mortality rates among seniors.[126]

Countries with high rates of consumption of dairy products and animal proteins also present the highest rates of bone fractures due to osteoporosis.[127] Two longitudinal studies (that is, studies that follow the subjects for many years) on women's health (one at Harvard University that followed 75,000 nurses over twelve years, and another in Sweden that involved 60,689 women over eleven years) found that an increase in milk consumption did not protect against the risk of osteoporotic fractures.[128] Also, two meta-analyses on the intake of milk or dairy products in relation to fracture risk did not report a drop in fracture risk with an increase in the intake of milk or dairy products or an increase in dietary calcium.[129]

Modern nutrition and osteoporosis

Contrary to primitive man's diet, which was largely based on foods such as fruits and wild plants, which are rich in alkaline substances, the Western diet is based on high consumption of meat, dairy products, cereals, sweets and salt, which leads to an excess acidity in the body that is not countered by a sufficient intake of alkaline foods such as fruits and vegetables. Blood pH levels outside alkaline values between 7.32 and 7.42 cannot sustain life. To protect itself from excess acidity (excess H^+ ions), the body has a buffer system that maintains normal pH levels in the blood. This buffer system introduces alkaline mineral substances such as calcium, magnesium and potassium, among others, into the bloodstream. These minerals are primarily found in bones and secondarily in other tissues such as cartilage, teeth and muscles.[130] The acid-base balance of body fluids is essential for the proper functioning of enzymatic reactions in the body, cellular metabolism, and oxygenation. In short, this balance is essential for homeostasis. Contributions in hydrogen ions—H^+ (acid intake)—derive from protein degradation and cell metabolism while contributions in HCO_3- (a molecule with a buffer role) are from alkaline foods such as vegetables.

The kidneys play an important role in this balance by allowing the removal of H^+ (acid molecules) and the reabsorption of HCO_3- (alkaline molecules).The acid-base balance is a very determinant factor in human health because it influences the structure and the function of proteins, the permeability of cellular membranes, the distribution of electrolytes and the structure of connective tissues.[131]

In young people, kidneys respond effectively to metabolic acidosis by increasing the excretion of H^+ ions, thereby minimizing blood pH perturbations.[132] However, our ability to excrete hydrogen ions decreases as we age—even for those of us in good health—and this drop becomes significant when we reach our fifties.[133] This implies that as the body ages, it increasingly acidifies, making it more and more necessary to increase the daily intake of fruits and vegetables. Fruits and vegetables have alkalinizing properties because they are metabolized in the form of bicarbonates (HCO_3), which not only help compensate for the drop in renal function but also protect this same function.[134]

Unfortunately, all surveys in North America show that most individuals have a low intake of fruits and vegetables. Because we continue to consume too much acidic food as we age, we develop a slow and gradual metabolic acidosis. (Metabolic acidosis occurs when the kidneys do not remove enough acid from the body.)

Because of that, demineralization and resorption of bones increase with age, thus favoring the onset of osteoporosis.[135] It's been shown that a diet rich in fruits and vegetables protects against osteoporosis because it leads to high mineral density of the femoral neck and a drop in biochemical markers for bone resorption in pre- and post-menopausal women.[136] Therefore, a high consumption of fruits and vegetables has a solidifying effect on bones; or at least, it helps them maintain their integrity, as the digestion of fruits and vegetables supplies a considerable amount of bicarbonate, an alkalinizing substance that prevents the body from drawing away alkaline salts in bones to maintain the slightly alkaline pH levels in the blood that are indispensable to life.

Lastly, the high consumption of sodium chloride or table salt (as is typically the case in a Western diet), along with an acidic diet, further increases the acidity of bodily fluids.[137] The effects of such a diet are amplified with age as kidney functions diminish, which could favor metabolic acidosis and the development of chronic diseases such as osteoporosis.[138] Relying on a number of scientific studies that show that a high consumption of dairy products does not protect adult women from fractures, the World Health Organization recommends an increase in physical activity, the reduction of salt and animal protein, and an increase in the consumption of fruits and vegetables to fight against osteoporosis.[139]

Calcium food sources

Even though an adequate intake of calcium cannot in itself prevent osteoporosis, it is nonetheless an indispensable mineral for healthy bones. Is it possible to efficiently replace dairy products as a source of calcium for bone development and still have healthy bones?

In Western countries, healthcare providers and nutritionists highly recommend dairy products for the growth and good health of bones. However, as we have seen, it's necessary to rethink this idea, given the long-term, adverse effects of the consumption of cow's milk and dairy products on human health. Many plants, such as green vegetables and legumes that are rich in fiber, antioxidants, micronutrients, vitamins and vegetable proteins, are excellent sources of calcium, and their consumption also helps to maintain a healthy body weight.[140] In addition, the calcium in plants tends to be easier to absorb than that from dairy products.[141] In fact, the calcium in legumes and most green vegetables is absorbed in humans in proportions of 40 percent to 64 percent compared to about 32 percent for calcium in milk.[142] The simple fact that one consumes the appropriate quantities of calcium and vitamin D does not lead to the optimum use of that calcium. A study of healthy teens showed that those on a Mediterranean diet had better rates of calcium absorption and retention, as well as a reduced urinal excretion of calcium,[143] even though they consumed less calcium compared to those on a Western diet. A diet such as the Mediterranean diet could lead to better bone growth and prevent diseases such as osteoporosis. It seems there is a positive link between the consumption of fruits and vegetables, which are abundant in the Mediterranean diet, and bone mineralization.[144]

List of foods containing interesting and bio-absorbable quantities of calcium

The following foods contain an interesting quantity of bio-absorbable calcium: some alkaline mineral waters rich in calcium (see chapter 6, section 2), firm tofu, enriched soy beverages, black-eyed peas, sesame seeds, almonds, parsley, flax seeds, chickpeas, dried apricots, dried figs, Chinese cabbage, kale, seaweed, white beans, kidney beans, arugula, sunflower seeds, sun-dried tomatoes, peanuts, currants, bok choy, broccoli, brussels sprouts, radishes, rutabaga.[145]

Daily calcium requirements

According to C.D. Hunt and L.K. Johnson,[146] our daily calcium requirements appear to be overestimated. In fact, according to R.P. Heaney,[147] for someone who eats adequately, calcium needs seem to be around 741 milligrams per day (mg/day) or even 500 mg/day, instead of 1200–1500 mg/day as generally suggested by nutritionists who rely on the recommendations provided by "Canada's Food Guide."[148] Hunt and Johnson's conclusions are based on the most extensive study available that consolidated calcium-balance data from metabolic studies that used the most controlled and rigorous experimental procedures.[149]

Osteoporosis and nutrition

Recent studies on bone health and the prevention of osteoporosis showed not only the importance of vitamin D[150] for good calcium absorption but also the contribution of minerals such as magnesium, potassium,[151] vitamin C,[152] vitamin K,[153] many B-complex vitamins and carotenoids.[154] Scientific studies that link the consumption of animal proteins and osteoporosis often have contradictory results. On the one hand, a high intake of animal proteins contributes to bone loss, but on the other hand, a low consumption of proteins has been linked to an increase in fracture risk in older individuals.[155]

In conclusion, it is obvious from numerous published studies that the best protection against osteoporosis is a balanced diet containing a large proportion of fruits and plants, reasonable consumption of animal proteins, moderate consumption of alcohol and limited consumption of foods containing empty calories such as sweets, farinaceous foods and foods classified as junk foods.[156] Such a diet, accompanied by regular physical exercise, significantly improves bone health in various age groups.[157] Nonetheless, in young[158] and menopausal women,[159] the acidity of body fluids could be buffered by the consumption of fruits and vegetables and the intake of an alkaline mineral water rich in calcium (= 200 milligrams per liter [mg/l]) and bicarbonate (= 1000 mg/l) and poor in sulfate (= 50 mg/l). In both groups, daily consumption of this kind of mineral water significantly reduces bone resorption.

7. COOKING FOOD
Seignalet and the hazards of cooking

According to Seignalet, as much as possible, foods should be eaten raw, as cooking very often leads to the formation of toxins due to the Maillard reaction. The Maillard reaction was described about a hundred years ago[160] by a French biochemist of the same name. During high-temperature cooking, principally of animal proteins and many cereals, the Maillard reaction causes changes in foods: color changes to yellowish brown, and odor and taste change in intensity. Since many foods require cooking before being eaten, one should try, as much as possible, to reduce both cooking temperature and cooking time. From 120°C (248°F), heat modifies the nature of proteins in the presence of carbohydrates (sugar), and these modifications can cause toxic and carcinogenic derivatives due to the creation of very strong chemical bonds, called covalent bonds, between carbohydrates and amino acids or proteins. These molecules are extremely complex, and our enzymes find it more and more difficult to digest them as they become more complex. The most complex molecules are insoluble in water and cannot be broken down by digestive enzymes.

In the presence of intestinal hyper-permeability, large molecules from the Maillard reaction can cross the intestinal barrier and accumulate if not in cells, then at the very least, in the extracellular medium, which in turn can lead to deposit pathologies. These molecules may also be captured by macrophages, which could transport them whole to areas of elimination, thus inducing elimination pathologies. Seignalet notes that where there is a heavy consumption of cooked animal meat, a heavy price is paid through obesity, type 2 diabetes, cardiovascular disease, breast cancer and colon cancer. Inuit peoples, who in the past ate mostly fish and raw caribou and also ate large quantities of animal fat, were usually ten times less likely to suffer from cardiovascular diseases compared to Europeans and Americans. Since they've adopted a Western-style diet, cardiovascular diseases and type 2 diabetes affect a large portion of the population.

Recent scientific studies confirming the harmfulness of some foods cooked at high temperatures

Recent scientific studies not only confirm Seignalet's assertions about the health hazards of high-temperature cooking, but even further highlight them, pointing out precisely the various mechanisms at work.

Cooking makes food molecules highly mobile, thus allowing new bonds to form between them. When amino acids, peptides or proteins react with sugar or lipids at high temperatures (110–180°C or 230–356°F), the Maillard reaction takes place, and new compounds form.[161] Different reaction products form when the Maillard reaction takes place without enzymes. In general, these products are called advanced glycation end-products (AGE) or glycotoxins.[162]

Dr. H. Vlassara's team has published more than 160 articles on glycotoxins and, in the early 1980s, was the first group to give priority to this area of research. There are various glycotoxins, but the Vlassara team concentrated particularly methylglyoxal (MG) and N-carboxymethyl-lysine (CML) derivatives. They based their quantification of the amount of glycotoxins in foods on the quantification of CML in more than 549 foods from 2003 to 2008.[163]

Glycotoxins and RAGE as catalysts of chronic disease

Glycotoxins have been categorized into five or even seven groups (depending on different studies), with each group presenting a different level of toxicity.[164] Maillard had already supposed that animal proteins modified in the Maillard reaction could play a role in chronic-disease pathology. This idea came up again about thirty years ago, and (mainly between 2003 and 2008) various research teams gave it special attention. Interest in the study of Maillard molecules has been rekindled thanks to the identification of a type of receptor on the cell surface referred to as the receptor for advanced glycation end-products or glycotoxins (RAGE).[165] In fact, the binding of glycotoxins to RAGEs on the cellular surface could activate a sequence of intracellular reactions that could increase oxidative stress, production of C-reactive proteins (CRP) and pro-inflammatory cytokines such as TNF-α.[166] Glycotoxins and their receptors may play a central role in inflammatory response and could be implicated in the aging process and in a number of chronic diseases linked to subclinical pre-symptomatic inflammation. The binding of glycotoxins to RAGEs could disturb cellular autoregulation functions as they become deposited on tissues, which (as shown by S. Bengmark) could lead to many diseases such as coronary disease, allergies, diabetes, Alzheimer's disease, rheumatoid arthritis, arthritis, cancers and kidney disease.[167] Since RAGE was only identified recently, many doctors and nutritionists do not yet know the negative effects of glycotoxins on health.

Correlation between the ingestion of glycotoxins, inflammation and life span

Studies on animals and humans have demonstrated that there is a significant correlation between ingestion of food glycotoxins, their presence in the bloodstream and the establishment of inflammation markers.[168] Earlier experiments on animals have already shown that on average, those that are fed sparingly lived twice as long as those that eat their fill.[169] However, the significance of these results was reconsidered following recently published studies showing that the increase in life span could be due to a drop in the quantity of ingested toxic substances, such as glycotoxins, and not due to the total quantity of calories ingested.[170] So, in animals, a diet low in glycotoxins but without any restriction on the number of calories ingested seems to increase life span just as a restriction in the amount of ingested calories would.

Similar observations were made in diabetic patients: those who followed a diet low in glycotoxins showed a considerable drop in inflammation markers and vascular dysfunction.[171] Also, the presence of glycotoxins in a diet is strongly associated with inflammation markers, oxidative stress and endothelial-cell dysfunction, not only in diabetic patients but also in normal subjects.[172] Many glycotoxins, such as acrylamide, are abundant in foods commonly consumed in a Western-type diet.[173]

Based on an analysis of the foods eaten in three days by ninety individuals in good health, it was found that an average American consumes about 16,000 ku, plus or minus 5,000 ku (kilo units per day, as determined by authors) of glycotoxins, and that such a diet significantly contributes to the pool of glycotoxins in the body.[174] This was further proven by the fact that a subgroup of the study in question, for which the consumption of dietary glycotoxins was reduced, experienced an average drop of serum glycotoxins of 30 percent to 40 percent.[175]

In general, only 10 percent of glycotoxins are absorbed by intestinal cells, and 30 percent of this value is excreted by the kidneys, while 70 percent is stored in various tissues.[176] Unfortunately, given that from age fifty, kidney efficiency drops even in healthy individuals, the effects of glycotoxin accumulation get worse with age. It is therefore no coincidence that in Western countries, chronic disease is increasingly frequent, particularly since the advent of industrialized food processing. A longitudinal study (one conducted over many years) on healthy, average elderly persons in Italy showed that the most significant factor linked to mortality was the drop in renal function. There could be an obvious link between inflammation, oxidizing stress, glycotoxins and chronic disease; and as a matter of fact, studies show that the incidence of chronic kidney disease as well as the cardiovascular diseases that develop with age could be lowered by reducing the level of glycotoxins in the diet either with the help of drugs or by ingesting fewer of them.[177]

Defense mechanisms against glycotoxins

Recent studies suggest that even though the amount of endogenous glycotoxins (those produced by the body) increases with age, dietary glycotoxins make up the majority of those found in the body and are responsible for age-related diseases.[178] Dietary glycotoxins are counted in milligrams, while endogenous glycotoxins present in biological systems could be counted in picograms; that is, a billion times less than dietary glycotoxins.[179]

Our bodies are naturally protected against the formation of endogenous glycotoxins by an enzymatic process: cell deglycation.[180] This process is an essential defense system in mammalian cells, but can go overboard in the case of diabetes due to hyperglycemia or of a chronic intake of excessive dietary glycotoxins, for example. It seems that another category of receptors that bind to glycotoxins—the AGE receptor-1 (AGER1)—has an antioxidant and anti-inflammatory action by inducing the degradation of glycotoxins. These receptors play a protective role, contrary to the RAGE, which activates inflammatory response.[181] A diet low in glycotoxins could favor an increase in AGER1 in tissues.[182]

There is some evidence that high levels of glycotoxins in an individual's diet have a direct influence on the quantity of glycotoxins in blood serum and in tissues, as well as on inflammation markers, leading to a drop in antioxidant reserves. It is possible to manage the amount of dietary glycotoxins, but if a high intake of glycotoxins is maintained, severe chronic diseases can develop as we age.[183]

Tissues most affected by glycotoxins

Non-soluble, non-digestible and dysfunctional glycotoxins accumulate mostly in collagen (a fibrous protein that is the main constituent of connective tissue) and myelin tissue (which forms a lipidic protective shield around nervous tissues). Their presence could explain the loss in elasticity that causes the age-dependent rigidity of tissues rich in collagen, such as the crystalline lens of the eye, joints, skeletal muscles and vascular walls.[184] A high consumption of foods that produce large quantities of glycotoxins when cooked at high temperature could contribute to a significant glycotoxin accumulation in these tissues. Tissues with a high concentration of glycotoxins caused by inadequate diet, as well as a growing number of RAGEs (as a consequence of the deposition of glycotoxins in tissues), are those that present a slow regeneration, as is the case for tendons, bones and the cartilage among others. The buildup of glycotoxins in these tissues could result in increased secretion of pro-inflammatory cytokines, which in the long run could lead to cellular dysfunction and the onset of disease.[185] Such changes could truly be responsible for the increase in rigidity and the weakening of structures such as intervertebral disks, tendons, cartilage, synovial membranes and skeletal muscles and could also be a major factor in the pathogenesis of arthritic diseases such as osteoarthritis, rheumatoid arthritis and fibromyalgia.[186] Recent in vitro and in vivo studies have highlighted the significant correlation between dietary glycotoxins and a number of disease risk factors, which supports the idea that a diet low in glycotoxins has promise as a therapeutic intervention.

Foods with a high glycotoxin content

The foods that contribute the most to the accumulation of glyco-toxins in human tissues are meats, especially if prepared at high temperatures. Depending on the manner of cooking (roasting, for example), the glycotoxin content of food can increase from four to nine times (in comparison with cooking by boiling—a better way to cook).[187] In general, fish contains ten times less glycotoxins than meat. The glycotoxin content is higher in milk powder in compari-son to fresh milk and could increase if the powder is kept at room temperature for many months. Milk powder contains thirty-six times more glycotoxins than raw milk and seven times more than pasteurized milk.[188] Dairy products in powder form are usually identified on their wrappings with terms such as "dairy products," "milk protein" or "dairy substances." For fresh milk (and not pow-dered milk), terms such as "pasteurized milk" or "raw milk" are clearly indicated, as in the case of some cheeses. So, powdered milk found in a good number of processed foods such as most ice creams, yogurts, baby formula and low-end cheeses and in fast foods such as pizzas, tacos, nachos and salad dressing could con-tain high levels of glycotoxins.[189] In the last decades, the food industry may even have added synthetic glycotoxins to foods in order to improve taste. As such, some mass-produced biscuits eas-ily contain up to 1,000 units of glycotoxins per biscuit.[190] Without any major prospective studies establishing nutritional guidelines on glycotoxin intake, it is difficult to determine the safe daily maxi-mum consumption with respect to criteria such as age and health status, to name just two. People who eat a diet rich in grilled or roasted meat, fats and industrially or commercially processed foods can easily consume 2,0000 ku[191] of glycotoxins per day.

Tables 4 and 5 indicate the levels of certain glycotoxins found in common foods.

TABLE 4: Quantification of carboxymethyl-lysine, a variety of glycotoxin in meat and fish[192]*

MEAT AND FISH	GLYCOTOXINS KU/100G
Raw beef	707
Roast beef	6,071
Grilled steak	7,479
Beef stew	2,657
Boiled chicken (1 hour)	1,123
Roast chicken: with BBQ sauce (skinless breast)	4,768
Fried chicken (20 minutes)	9,722
Chicken: dark meat, roasted (15 minutes)	8,299
Potted chicken: cooked in liquid (1 hour)	3,329
Chicken: fast food nuggets	8,627
Chicken: with skin, roasted on BBQ, sauce added at the end	18,520
Pork: bacon, fried without added oil (5 minutes)	91,577
Pork: bacon, microwaved, 2 slices (3 minutes)	9,023
Pork chops: marinated in balsamic vinegar, BBQ	3,334
Sausages, beef and pork: pan-fried	5,426
Boiled lamb (30 minutes)	1,218
Roast lamb, 450°F/230°C (30 minutes)	2,431
Veal stew	2,858
Boiled or poached fish	761
Atlantic salmon: poached, medium heat (7 minutes)	1,801
Smoked salmon	572
Grilled salmon with olive oil	4,334
Salmon: cooked in a pan with olive oil	3,083
Fried shrimp (to go)	4,328
Fresh tuna: cooked (25 minutes)	919
Canned tuna in water	452
Canned tuna in oil	1,740
Big Mac	7,801

*   N.B.: These values indicate only the amounts from carboxymethyl-lysine's glyco-toxins and therefore do not take into account other glycotoxins such as methylglyoxal or acrylamide and other varieties that could be found in food.

TABLE 5: Quantities of carboxymethyl-lysine in various common foods[193]*

FOOD	GLYCOTOXINS KU/100G
Brie	5,597
Cheddar	5,523
Parmesan cheese (Kraft)	16,900
Soy burger	67–437
Grilled tofu	4,107
Firm raw tofu	788
Soft raw tofu	488
Boiled tofu, 5 minutes	628–796
Fried eggs	2,749
Omelet: low temperature, oil sprayed (11 minutes)	90
Omelet: with margarine (8 minutes)	163
Omelet: with butter (13 minutes)	507
Omelet: with olive oil (12 minutes)	337
Poached eggs (5 minutes)	90
Biscuits (McDonald's)	1,470
Legumes	Less than 300
Cereal bar	507–3,177
Commercial biscuits	500–1,800
Commercial donuts (Krispy Kreme)	1,400–1,800
All fresh fruits	Less than 50
Dried fruit other than figs	Less than 170
Dried figs	2,663
Raw vegetables	Less than 130
Grilled vegetables	Less than 262
Soup: with or without meat	Less than 2

* N.B. These values contain only the amounts from carboxymethyl-lysine's glyco-toxins and do not take into account other glycotoxins such as methylglyoxal or acrylamide that could be found in food.

Acrylamide: A particularly toxic glycotoxin
produced during the cooking of some foods

The Maillard reaction leads to the formation of some intermediary products, depending on the components present in some foods. These, in turn, produce some glycotoxins that have various levels of toxicity. Acrylamide[194] is a particularly harmful glycotoxin, long known for its neurotoxicity (that is, its toxic action on the nervous system). It's used in medical research but is handled with great caution. Acrylamide could disrupt the transport of essential substances to axons (the nerve fiber that carries nervous impulses) and cause degeneration.[195] It was only in 2002, and mostly by chance, that Dr. Margareta Törnqvist's Swedish research team discovered the presence of a large quantity of acrylamide (150–4,000 micrograms per kilogram [4,000 µg/kg]) in foods cooked at high temperatures, such as bread, biscuits, fried potatoes and chips.[196] At first, these results were refuted and described as fearmongering, but researchers from Britain, Norway and Switzerland obtained similar results with cereals (grains), chips, fries and biscuits.[197] Since then, because of its known toxic influence on the nervous system, and owing to the place occupied in the Western diet by some of the foods containing particularly high amounts of it, acrylamide in food has been the subject of many studies. During a Maillard reaction, foods that contain high quantities of asparagine (an amino acid) and sugar (starch), as is the case with potatoes and a majority of wheat-related grains, produce acrylamide when cooked at temperatures higher than 110°C (230°F).[198] When foods containing carbohydrates and lipids are cooked at high temperatures, other glycotoxins, such as carboxymethyl-lysine and methylglyoxal, are produced during a reaction between these carbohydrates and lipids and the amino acids lysine and arginine.[199]

Table 6 shows the daily consumption in the U.S. of plant-based foods, rich in asparagine, cooked at high temperatures and containing acrylamide.[200]

TABLE 6: Daily consumption of foods rich in asparagine and containing acrylamide

FOOD	ACRYLAMIDE (µG/KG)	CONSUMPTION (µG/KG)
White bread	11	0.29–0.77
Whole-wheat bread	39	0.43–2.38
Ready-to-eat cereals	86	1.99–4.88
Wheaten cereals	738	30.3
Toasted bread	213	1.64–7.31
Coffee	7	1.71–3.73
Crackers (all types)	188	2.37–7.76
Graham crackers	459	5.78–19
Tortillas	199	0.80–9.15
Fries	413	5–26.3
Olives (canned)	414	0.28–4.14
Peanut butter	88	0.31–2.99
Popcorn	180	0.47–4.32
Chips	466	2.47–14.4
Postum (a coffee alternative made with wheat)	4,573	0.01–13.7

A study[201] carried out by the state of California revealed that Americans get 38 percent of their acrylamide from their consumption of fried potatoes, 17 percent from cookies, cakes and crackers, 14 percent from bread, 9 percent from cereal-derived products (pastas, ready-to-eat cereals, etc.), 8 percent from coffee and 14 percent from other foods.

Significantly, the origin and conditions of plant cultivation can have a great impact on the concentration of acrylamide in food. For example, chips made from potatoes grown in Korea have an acrylamide concentration that varies from 408 to 3,241 µg/kg. Variation in the quantities of acrylamide found in a particular food could be due not only to cultivars but also to growth methods (use of fertilizers, etc.), harvesting methods and conditions during processing, such as pH levels, storage temperature and duration of exposure to heat.[202]

Methods for reducing the levels of acrylamide in food

There are many ways to potentially reduce the harmful effects of acrylamide in the industrialized mass-production of food:[203]

1) Select varieties of potato plants that contain lower levels of asparagine, a precursor of acrylamide.
2) Remove asparagine in the first step of the industrial preparation.
3) Use the enzyme asparaginase to hydrolyze asparagine into aspartic acid to prevent acrylamide formation.
4) Select procedures that minimize acrylamide formation by adjusting pH levels, temperature, length of cooking time and storage conditions.
5) Add substances to food that can prevent acrylamide formation, such as antioxidants, acidifying substances such as lemon juice and vinegar, some amino acids and sugars that do not react with asparagine.
6) Remove acrylamide after its formation with some purification methods.

Our government authorities are fully aware of the dangers of acrylamide in our food and are trying to minimize its importance, as indicated by the information a Health Canada representative gave on the TV show *L'Épicerie* in 2003. Fortunately, some important information on acrylamide was also provided during this show. You can find this program (in French) at www.radio-canada.ca/actualite/lepicerie/docArchives/2003/03/21/enquete.html.

People's health will continue to deteriorate, and chronic diseases will continue to be a burden on our public health system as long as the public is kept ignorant of the dangers of acrylamide and other glycotoxins, and no pressure is exerted on government institutions to prompt the food industry to make changes.

Cooking and its influence on the formation
of mutagen molecules

It has now been established that cooking foods at temperatures higher than 110°C (230°F) contributes to the acceleration of the aging process and the onset of many chronic diseases. A high concentration of some molecules from the Maillard reaction may also have some mutagenic effects (that is, gene modification).[204] There is increasing evidence that indicates that glycotoxin receptors—RAGEs—could play a determinant role in the development of cancers.[205] The presence of these receptors increases with the amount of glycotoxin in tissues. In cancer cells, RAGEs were linked, for a variety of tumor types, to an increase in metastasis and worsening of patients' physiological state. These receptors can interact by directly activating cancer cells and stimulating their proliferation, their invasion abilities, the formation of metastasis, their angiogenesis (development of new blood vessels to feed tumors) and their chemo resistance (resistance to specific treatment).[206]

How you, personally, can resolve the cooking issue

To resolve the issue of Maillard-molecule formation, Dr. Seignalet advised that foods be eaten raw. However, if you want to eat cooked foods, you must take into account the fact that modifications induced by heat are proportional to the temperature and the cooking time. The temperature from which food starts to undergo noticeable transformation is around 110°C (230°F). In fact, Dr. Seignalet was inspired by the works of Dr. Catherine Kousmine,[207] who recommended avoiding grilling and frying, which occur at temperatures close to 300°C (575°F) and 700°C (1300°F). Dr. Kousmine advised that food should mostly be gently steamed. According to her, one should consider the fact that foods with mainly animal proteins produce more Maillard molecules than carbohydrate foods. Adding fat increases the production of glycotoxins.

Recent studies show that the majority of AGE or glycotoxins are found mainly in foods containing proteins from animals and cereals and cooked at high temperatures,[208] which includes frying, barbecuing and grilling. Glycotoxin levels are even higher in processed foods such as deli meats, bacon, powdered egg whites and powdered milk, which are based on animal products. Cooking temperature seems to have more impact than cooking time, and debates continue about the harmfulness of microwave cooking for all foods. According to some, microwave cooking increases the amount of glycotoxins faster than classic cooking methods.[209] When it comes to cooking vegetables, the preservation of nutrients in foods is mostly the issue, as vegetables contain very few glycotoxins. Here again, there is no consensus on microwave cooking, and the debate is mostly about the power level used, the cooking time and the amount of water added. It is, however, generally accepted that the more water that is added to vegetables, the greater the amount of nutrients that leak into the cooking water.

The consumption of glycotoxins cannot be totally avoided, but by changing our cooking methods, we can at least reduce the amount we ingest. Foods that are likely to contain a non-negligible quantity of glycotoxins are best steamed, boiled, poached, cooked at a lower temperature in a liquid, stir-fried or cooked in a slow cooker in a liquid at low temperature. These methods allow not only for low-temperature cooking, but also for the retention of liquids. Research has shown that, to a great extent, water and other liquids inhibit the formation of glycotoxins during cooking.[210] In conclusion, remember that simple changes in our cooking habits can prevent a great number of chronic diseases associated with inflammation stemming from toxin accumulation in some foods cooked at high temperatures (110°C to 180°C, or 230°F to 356°F).

8. UPDATE FROM THE LATEST SCIENTIFIC PUBLICATIONS: LINKS BETWEEN "LEAKY GUT," THE MODERN GLYCOTOXIN-RICH DIET AND CHRONIC INFLAMMATORY DISEASE

By Jean-Yves Dionne, BSc. Pharm., lecturer and
consultant in natural health products

The permeability of the small intestine is regulated by zonulin proteins, which modulate intercellular tight junctions, the key structures that allow paracellular trafficking of macromolecules. The up-regulation of zonulin proteins causes an increase in small intestinal permeability and may lead to immune-mediated diseases.[1]

Until the late 1980s, the small intestine was described as a tube composed of a single layer of cells (enterocytes) that connected to each other via the tight junctions. In addition to digestion and absorption, the tight junctions were thought to keep all but the smallest molecules away from the components of the immune system in underlying tissues.

The theory that a "leaky gut" contributes to immune-mediated diseases[2] was initially greeted with skepticism, partly because of the way that scientists thought of the intestines. The discovery of zonulin proteins, the only known physiological modulator of intercellular tight junctions described so far, allows for a better understanding of the mechanisms regulating gut permeability.[3] The interplays between environmental factors, specific susceptibility genes, zonulin proteins and the tight junctions underlie the aberrant immune response that influences the reaction to nonself antigens. When the zonulin pathway is deregulated in genetically susceptible individuals exposed to environmental triggers, immune disorders can occur because the integrity of the intestinal barrier is compromised.[4] The role of zonulin proteins subverts traditional theories regarding the development of immune-mediated diseases and suggests that these processes can be arrested if environmental triggers (gluten, for example) can be avoided. For example, in celiac disease patients (except in rare cases), once gluten is removed from the diet, serum zonulin levels decrease, the intestine resumes its baseline barrier functions, auto-antibody titers are normalized, the autoimmune process stops and intestinal damage heals completely.[4]

In brief, genetic predisposition, miscommunication between innate and adaptive immunity, exposure to environmental triggers and zonulin-dependent loss of intestinal barrier function causing a dysfunction of the intercellular tight junctions all seem to be key ingredients in the pathogenesis of several immune and/or autoimmune diseases. This theory implies that once the autoimmune process is activated, it is not auto-perpetuating. The continuous stimulation by nonself antigens (environmental triggers) seems to be necessary to perpetuate the process.[4] Rather, the autoimmune process can be modulated or even reversed by preventing the continual interplay between genes and environmental triggers.

Moreover, this model suggests that new therapeutic strategies aimed at reestablishing intestine-barrier function offer innovative and hitherto unexplored approaches for the management of many other devastating chronic diseases. Already, the zonulin pathway has been exploited to facilitate delivery of drugs and antigens through several epithelial and endothelial barriers, thus allowing the passage of therapeutic agents into/through the gastrointestinal tract, the airways and the blood-brain barrier.[5]

Recent works suggest and/or demonstrate the possible role of the small intestine hyper-permeability, together with an increase of zonulin proteins, in many immune-mediated diseases: obesity and obesity-associated insulin resistance, autoimmune diseases like ankylosing spondylitis, inflammatory bowel disease (Crohn's disease), rheumatoid arthritis, systemic lupus erythematosus, type 1 diabetes; cancers such as brain cancers (gliomas), breast cancer, lung adenocarcinoma, ovarian cancer, pancreatic cancer; and diseases of the nervous system such as chronic inflammatory demyelinating polyneuropathy, multiple sclerosis andschizophrenia.[1,5,6,7]

Environmental triggers play an essential role in the development of immune-mediated diseases. According to Dr. Seignalet, the consumption of large amounts of glycotoxins (advanced glycation end products) in modern alimentation, mostly from animal proteins and wheat grains cooked at high temperatures (Maillard's reaction) may act as predominant triggers in chronic inflammatory diseases.

Since 2003, we've known that receptors for glycotoxins—RAGES— play a key role in the development and progression of chronic inflammatory diseases. Because RAGE receptors can bind glycotoxins deposited in the tissues, they can modify the structure, function and mechanical properties of tissues through crosslinking intracellular as well as extracellular matrix proteins. The role of glycotoxins (AGEs) and glycotoxin receptors (RAGES), as well as leaky gut, is well demonstrated in many diseases: diabetes mellitus, cancers, Alzheimer's disease, rheumatoid arthritis, osteoarthritis, cardiovascular and renal diseases.[6,7,8,9,10,11,12,13,14,15,16,17,18,19]

REFERENCES

1. A. Fasano, "Intestinal permeability and its regulation by zonulin: Diagnostic and therapeutic implications," *Clin Gastroenterol Hepatol,* vol. 10, 2012, p. 1096–1100.

2. I. Bjarnason, T.J. Peters, N. Veall N. et al., "Intestinal permeability defect in celiac disease," *Lancet,* vol. 1, 1983, p. 1284–85.

3. A. Fasano, T. Not, W. Wang et al., "zonulin, a newly discovered modulator of intestinal permeability, and its expression in celiac disease," *Lancet,* vol. 355, 2000, p. 1518–19.

4. A. Fasano, "Leaky gut and autoimmune diseases," *Clinic Rev Allerg Immunol,* vol. 42, 2012, p. 71–78.

5. K.H. Song, N.D. Eddington, "The impact of AT1002 on the delivery of ritonavir in the presence of bioadhesive polymer, carrageenan," *Arch Pharm Res,* vol. 35, 2012, p. 937–43.

6. S. de Kort, D. Keszthelyi, A.A. Masclee, "Leaky gut and diabetes mellitus: What is the link?" *Obes Rev,* vol. 12, 2011, p. 449–58. Review.

7. J.M. Moreno-Navarrete, M. Sabater, F. Ortega et al., "Circulating zonulin, a marker of intestinal permeability, is increased in association with obesity-associated insulin resistance," PLoS One, 7(5):e37160. Epub 2012 May 18.

8. A.M. Yaser, Y. Huang, R.R. Zhou et al., "The role of receptor for advanced glycation end products (RAGE) in the proliferation of hepatocellular carcinoma," *Int J Mol Sci,* vol. 13, 2012, p. 5982–97.

9. D. Carnevale, G. Mascio, I. D'Andrea et al., "Hypertension induces brain β-amyloid accumulation, cognitive impairment, and memory deterioration through activation of receptor for advanced glycation end products in brain vasculature," *Hypertension,* vol. 60, 2012, p. 188–97.

10. J. Todorova, E. Pasheva, "High mobility group B1 protein interacts with its receptor RAGE in tumor cells but not in normal tissues," *Oncol Lett,* vol. 3, 2012, 214–18.

11. S. Mizumoto, J. Takahashi, K. Sugahara, "Receptor for advanced glycation end products (RAGE) functions as receptor for specific sulfated glycosaminoglycans, and anti-RAGE antibody or sulfated glycosaminoglycans delivered in vivo inhibit pulmonary metastasis of tumor cells," *J Biol Chem.,* vol. 287, 2012, p. 18985–94.

12. S. Gangemi, A. Allegra, M. Aguennouz et al. "Relationship between advanced oxidation protein products, advanced glycation end products, and S-nitrosylated proteins with biological risk and MDR-1 polymorphisms in patients affected by B-chronic lymphocytic leukemia," *Cancer Invest,* 2012, 30:20–26.

13. I. Elangovan, S. Thirugnanam, A. Chen et al., "Targeting receptor for advanced glycation end products (RAGE) expression induces apoptosis and inhibits prostate tumor growth," *Biochem Biophys Res Commun.,* vol. 417, 2012, p. 1133–38.

14. S. Grimm, C. Ott, M. Hörlacher, "Advanced glycation end products-induced formation of immunoproteasomes: involvement of the receptor for AGEs and Jak2/STAT1," *Biochem J.* 2012, Aug 15. [Epub ahead of print].

15. D.J. Leong, H.B. Sun, "Events in articular chondrocytes with aging," *Curr Osteoporos,* vol. 9, 2011, p. 196–201. Review.

16. H. Hiraiwa, T. Sakai, H. Mitsuyama et al., "Inflammatory effect of advanced glycation end products on human meniscal cells from osteoarthritic knees," *Inflamm Res,* vol. 60, 2011, p. 1039–48.

17. K. Takada, J. Hirose, K. Senba et al., "Enhanced apoptotic and reduced protective response in chondrocytes following endoplasmic reticulum stress in osteoarthritic cartilage," *Int J Exp Pathol,* vol. 92, 2011, p. 232–42.

18. I. Makulska, M. Szczepańska, D. Drożdż et al., "Skin autofluorescence as a marker of cardiovascular risk in children with chronic kidney disease," 2012 Sep 15. [Epub ahead of print]

19. L.S. Tam, Q. Shang, E.K. Li et al., "Serum soluble receptor for advanced glycation end products levels and aortic augmentation index in early rheumatoid arthritis: A prospective study," *Semin Arthritis Rheum,* 2012 Aug 21. [Epub ahead of print].

5

BASIC PRINCIPLES OF
THE HYPOTOXIC DIET

1. POTENTIAL BENEFITS AND
MAIN REQUIREMENTS

Dr. Seignalet's diet is referred to as the ancestral, hypotoxic or original-type diet, and these terms are interchangeable. The diet is intended primarily for those who suffer from chronic inflammatory diseases, especially "arthritic diseases," a term that designates hundreds of conditions. If followed faithfully, this diet has the potential to produce three benefits:

1) The disappearance of chronic and intolerable ailments
2) Recovery of normal physical capabilities, such as the ability to use hands and legs without pain
3) Recovery of a normal quality of life

Secondarily, his diet is also meant for people in their fifties or older who have noticed (as the years go by) that they have stiffness in their hands and increasing pain when they walk. And finally, everyone should be aware of the particular dangers of certain foods and limit their consumption of these items.

The primary objective of the hypotoxic diet is to make sure that we consume only those foods that are appropriate and exclude from our diet all foods that are inappropriate and/or dangerous. According to Seignalet, if foods are of good quality, the issue of quantity becomes irrelevant; however, it is always better to eat less than to eat too much.

The diet's main requirements are the following:

1) Exclusion of animal milk of all origins and all its derivatives.

2) Exclusion of cereals, essentially wheat, barley, rye, oats and corn and all related cereals. Rice, buckwheat and sesame are allowed.

3) Exclusion of products cooked at high temperatures (that is, above 110°C [230°F]). Very few mutagenic and Maillard molecules form when foods are cooked below this temperature.

4) Exclusion of meat cooked at high temperatures.

5) Exclusion of refined oils, replacing them with unheated virgin oils.

6) Lowest possible consumption of polluted products and, by implication, a high consumption of organic foods.

7) Lowest possible consumption of processed foods.

8) Lowest possible consumption of refined white sugar.

9) Limited consumption of salt.

The Paleolithic diet experience

Recently, a team of American researchers attempted to verify if a diet close to that of our hunter-gatherer ancestors, who lived before the agricultural era, had any health benefits.[1] Nine volunteers, who were sedentary, not obese and in good health (which was verified by various tests), first followed their usual diet for three days. They were then subjected to a Mediterranean-style diet (meat, fish, chicken, eggs, fruits, milk products, vegetables, cereals, grains, apples, nuts, canola oil, mayonnaise and honey) for seven days; and next they followed a "Paleolithic" diet (lean meat, fish, eggs, fruits, vegetables, natural nuts, canola oil, mayonnaise and honey) for ten days. Excluded from the Paleolithic diet were milk products, legumes and cereals. To prevent any weight loss, special attention was paid to the quantity of food eaten, and the diet was adjusted accordingly. Foods in the Paleolithic diet were cooked by employees of the clinical research center. A number of tests were carried out to evaluate the effects of the different diets on the physiological state of the participants:

1) Measurement of blood pressure
2) Evaluation of the excretion of sodium and potassium (every twenty-four hours)
3) Evaluation of glucose and insulin during an oral glucose tolerance test (done two hours after the meal), and blood analysis to determine the speed at which sugar was eliminated from the blood
4) Evaluation of sensitivity to insulin
5) Evaluation of plasmatic concentration of lipid
6) Responsiveness of the brachial artery (artery in the arms) to ischemia (indicator of cardiovascular risk)

A comparison of these three diets showed that only the Paleolithic diet caused a significant drop in blood pressure and great elasticity of the arteries; a significant drop in plasmatic insulin as a function of time during the oral glucose tolerance test; a pronounced drop in the total levels of cholesterol in the blood, low-density lipoproteins (LDL) ("bad" cholesterol); and the presence of triglycerides in eight of the nine participants. The authors concluded that even a short-term Paleolithic diet in a ten-day period had improved blood pressure glucose tolerance, and caused a drop in the secretion of insulin, an increase in insulin sensitivity and an improvement in the lipid profile without loss of weight in sedentary humans in good health.

2. ANALYSIS OF VARIOUS FOODS
Animal milk

Animal milk (cow, goat, lamb, horse and others) and its derivatives— butter, cheese, cream, ice cream and yogurt—are forbidden on the hypotoxic diet. Contrary to popular belief, eliminating milk products from the diet does not lead to calcium deficiency. According to Seignalet, there are two reasons for this:

1) Animal milk, especially cow's milk, is very rich in calcium. However, only a small portion of the calcium is absorbed by the human small intestine. The rest is precipitated in the form of calcium phosphate, which is insoluble and is eliminated in the stool.
2) Calcium is available in sufficient quantities in vegetables, legumes, raw vegetables and fruits.

Grains

Seignalet considers proteins from most grains dangerous because they are always cooked at high temperatures, and our bodies' digestive enzymes are not able to effectively digest these foods, which became a part of our diet only 10,000 years ago. Whole-wheat bread is even worse than classic white bread as it is richer in Maillard molecules. As a matter of fact, Seignalet was right in saying whole-wheat bread contained more Maillard molecules than white bread, as we now know that the amino acid asparagine, which along with sugar is responsible for acrylamide formation after cooking at high temperatures, is more concentrated on the skin of the grain used in making whole-wheat bread.[2] In fact, one must eliminate from one's diet all products that contain wheat flour or wheat-related flour, such as rye, which is even richer in asparagine,[3] kamut, spelt, barley and oats. Even beer containing proteins from barley had a negative effect on some of Dr. Seignalet's patients. Corn is dangerous for the same reasons: thus, cornflakes, popcorn, kernels of sweet corn and corn flour must be eliminated, too. Significantly, in trying to determine which foods are responsible for inflammatory diseases, studies show that milk products, grains (especially the large family of wheat) and corn are at the top of the list.[4]

Also, according to Dr. Seignalet, rice has remained in its prehistoric form, and experiments have shown that it is seldom harmful. Therefore, white and brown rice are allowed. In fact, it's been established that the consumption of rice is safe mainly due to it containing very little or no free asparagine, the amino acid responsible for acrylamide production in the presence of carbohydrates (sugar), which is found in grains and certain plants cooked at high temperatures.[5] (As an aside, rice flour contains no glutens.) The fact that very little free asparagine was found in rice explains why cooking it leads to little or no acrylamide production, and eating it has no harmful effects on older individuals or on those genetically predisposed to inflammatory diseases.

Buckwheat is allowed because it is not graminaceous and it is generally well tolerated by most people. However, a non-negligible percentage of people are allergic to or intolerant of buckwheat,[6] so it's imperative to be careful when consuming it, particularly if one is already sensitive to some cereal proteins. Buckwheat has many interesting characteristics: it does not contain gluten and is rich in rutin. Rutin has antioxidant, anti-inflammatory and anti-cancerous properties. It is a very powerful natural inhibitor of the formation of glycotoxins produced during Maillard reactions,[7] which is why this cereal is well tolerated. Sesame is generally well tolerated by most people and contains antioxidants that favor the prevention of diseases linked to old age.[8] Dr. Seignalet made no comment regarding African cereals (millets and sorghum) as he knew nothing about them. According to him, the danger lies in mutated and cooked proteins. Finally, as carbohydrates are not harmful, the presence of cornstarch or wheat syrup in a product should not be a problem.

Meat and animal proteins

Dr. Seignalet considers that meat is bad when eaten cooked but good when eaten raw. Since not everyone can eat raw meat, he recommends that it be cooked at very low temperatures and for the shortest possible time. Lean meats are preferable because they do not usually contain large quantities of lipophilic waste as fatty meats do. Cooked meats (like sausages) should be avoided. He recommends that eggs be eaten raw or hard boiled at very low temperatures, or as runny omelets. For Seignalet, gently steamed fish is less dangerous than cooked meat. This fact was later confirmed by many studies.[9] Crustaceans are allowed.

Vegetables, legumes and fruits

All vegetables are allowed. Those that need to be cooked must be gently steamed. The following raw vegetables are recommended: garlic, carrots, celery, mushrooms, cucumbers, squash, watercress, endive, mache (leaves of genus *Valerianella* used in salad), melons, onions, peppers, radishes, green lettuce and tomatoes. Boiled or steamed dried vegetables or legumes are allowed: fava beans, white or red beans, lentils, sweet potatoes, peas, chickpeas, potatoes, quinoa, soy and tapioca. Soy milk and soy yogurt can be taken in moderation (see chapter 6, section 1). All fresh fruits are highly recommended. Dried or canned fruits are well represented in the diet: almonds, peanuts, dates, figs, hazelnuts, walnuts, olives, pine nuts and prunes. They should be eaten raw.

Sugars

White sugar must be avoided and replaced with brown sugar, which is richer in potassium, magnesium, calcium, phosphorus, iron and vitamins. Seignalet states that in one participant following the pre-historic diet, the endocrine pancreas and target organs of insulin were free from grime. Consequently, a reasonable intake of brown sugar would lead to a physiological insulin response that maintains glucose at an acceptable level. To replace bread and pasta as slow-to-digest sugars, he recommends the fructose found in fruits as the sugar with the slowest metabolism. In a body free of grime (such as the participant's mentioned above), the liver can easily draw from its glycogen and fatty-acids reserves to provide glucose on demand. As far as bread and pasta are concerned, it is now possible to find bread and pasta made of white or brown rice—and these are usually very good.

Oils

According to Seignalet, all refined oils and margarines are prohibited. This, however, does not apply to some new brands of margarine that do not contain hydrogenated oils (see chapter 6, section 8). Conversely, it is proper to say that raw virgin oils should be part of the diet. Seignalet recommends the following oils: a) olive oil containing monosaturated fatty acids; b) raw nuts oils, rapeseed oil that provides alpha-linolenic acid; c) primrose and borage oils that provide gamma-linoleic acid. Many other oils are acceptable, provided they are virgin and are consumed raw. The "virgin" indication means that the oil was extracted from the plant using only manual or mechanical processes and that it was not heated or subjected to any chemical treatment.

Virgin oils must meet the following criteria: a) extraction by mechanical processes only; b) clarification using only manual or mechanical processes; c) no chemical processing or refining; d) no use of insecticides or pesticides. Virgin oils are fragile and unstable in air, light and heat. They should be kept in brown bottles or metallic containers and refrigerated once they are opened.

Other foods

The following are allowed: honey, pollen, germinated legume seeds or unmutated ancestral cereals (soybeans, lentils, chickpeas, beans, alfalfa and rice). Cooked chocolate containing refined sugars should be consumed only in very small quantities. Dark, organic chocolate with brown sugar is preferable. Cooked jams full of white sugar should be avoided. All condiments are allowed: natural salts—like Himalayan salt, which is rich in minerals and oligoelements— peppers, vinegar, lemons, onions, garlic, mustard, parsley, capers, pickles, curry and aromatic plants. Salt should be used sparingly.

Beverages

Drinks rich in white sugar and beer containing barley proteins should be excluded. Allowable drinks include tap water and various mineral waters. Coffee and tea should be consumed within reason. Chicory is encouraged because of its choleretic properties (production of bile by the kidneys) and its depurative properties (waste elimination). Alcoholic beverages other than beer are allowed in moderation. Dr. Seignalet recommends that caution be used in the consumption of soy milk.

3. HOW I ADAPTED TO THE HYPOTOXIC DIET

As I mentioned in chapter 2, I went on the hypotoxic diet in June 2007. At the very beginning, I eliminated all milk products and cereals except for rice, buckwheat and sesame seeds. To maximize the diet's effects, I kept away from eggs and all sorts of nuts, which usually caused me trouble if I ate them more than once or twice a month.

For cooking, one can replace milk with non-dairy beverages made from soybeans, rice or almonds. Cream can be replaced with a creamy soybean preparation. I am satisfied with these substitutes as I find that they do not change the taste of food. It was, however, more complicated to replace bread. At the beginning, I was able to find (at the store) bread made from brown rice that was vacuum sealed and kept at room temperature. This bread was hard and barely acceptable when toasted. At first, I replaced wheat pasta with rice pasta. These changes in my diet resulted in a total disappearance, within ten days, of the unbearable pain in my hands and strongly motivated me to continue following the hypotoxic diet to the letter.

Later on, in an attempt to replace the vacuum-sealed bread that I didn't like, I tried different bread recipes with different types of flour—buckwheat, brown rice, tapioca—in different combinations, with some success (to say the least). I also made pancakes from buckwheat flour to replace the toast. After some time, I realized that I had developed an intolerance to buckwheat, which manifested in headaches that, in turn, disappeared in two days when I stopped eating buckwheat. This experience once more showed me how necessary it is to pay attention when introducing new foods into one's diet, especially if one has a history of intolerance to certain foods. There are many commercial types of bread that suit the hypotoxic diet. There is also a recipe for brown-rice bread on my blog (jacquelinelagace.net) (French only). Later tests caused me to conclude that I could not eat quinoa pasta and millet cereals. Moreover, chia grains, recommended for their richness in short-chain omega-3 fatty acids, had the same negative effects on me as had whole wheat. You must consider personal intolerances to certain foods and pay close attention to personal reactions when introducing new foods into your diet, even if these foods seem not to have any links to foods prohibited by the hypotoxic diet.

Given the benefits I enjoyed as a result of the hypotoxic diet, I always tried my best, even though I did not always succeed, to eat vegetables raw or to cook them just by slow steaming (as opposed to cooking presto). I also considerably reduced my consumption of red meat and grilled meat. I try to limit myself to one portion of meat per day. Of course, as much as possible, I avoid sweets and junk food.

It is not always easy to follow the hypotoxic diet. The beginning is especially difficult. That's why one day, after being on the hypotoxic diet for about two months, I ate 300 milliliters of commercial yogurt—which rekindled the intense pain in my metacarpophalangeal joints for the next two days. A few times during my first month on the diet, I drifted a little by eating hard-wheat spaghetti. On each occasion, on the following night, I felt very unpleasant pressure in the joints at the base of my fingers, but nothing compared to the pain that had followed the consumption of the yogurt.

I went through a very revealing experience in October 2007. One day, I ate quinoa spaghetti topped with a homemade tomato sauce and soybean cheese. The following night, I woke up to a sharp pain in the joint at the base of my right thumb. At first I wondered if the problem could have been caused by the quinoa. Then, as I read through the list of ingredients in the soybean cheese, I noticed that the cheese contained milk proteins. This experience illustrates how necessary it is to always check the list of ingredients in any food if you wish to avoid foods that are harmful to you.

After following the diet for three months, my sleep became much better. When I woke up during the night, I was able to go back to sleep right away—unlike before, when it would take me three to four hours to go back to sleep. I also gradually started recovering the partial use of my hands. I could once more bend my thumb metacarpophalangeal joints, but I still could not fold them at the terminal phalangeal joint. Also, my ring fingers, which I could not bend to an angle lower than 90 degrees before I started the diet, could now bend to about a 45 degree angle. I still was unable to close my hands, but I was very much encouraged by the results I'd obtained within the first three months of the diet.

During the months that followed, the joints on my hands gradually recovered their flexibility, so much so that in October 2008—sixteen months after I began the hypotoxic diet—I was able to completely close my hands. Nonetheless, I had sustained some light injury in the little finger and ring finger on my right hand. Even though they bend well, and even though I can close my hand completely, these two fingers do not close as completely as the index and middle fingers. If I refer to Dr. Seignalet's theory, it appears that my recovery of the use of the joints on my fingers results from the fact that the hypotoxic diet has gradually cleansed these joints, allowing them to recover their capacity to bend. Because, in general, the tissues had not yet been totally destroyed by my chronic inflammatory disease but only blocked by the accumulation of toxic molecules from the small intestines (macro-molecules from bacteria and food), a return to normal was possible. However, it seems that for the little finger and the ring finger on my right hand, the joint tissues must have suffered some degree of permanent damage, so much so that I am not able to bend these two fingers fully.

During the first year, I rigorously followed the hypotoxic diet with very little divergence. I drifted only when I was invited to eat at a friend's house or when we went out to a restaurant. I did not want to impose my diet on others during such occasions, and of course, from time to time, I also appreciated the short break. Usually, this didn't happen more than once a week; and I either did not feel any negative effects or felt only very minor effects when I occasionally diverged.

When I travel, even though certain foods are unavoidable, I try not to eat any dairy products and products from grains, but I also avoid being overzealous by asking for the detailed contents of the meal. It does happen sometimes—occasionally, though—that I'll eat white bread and wheat spaghetti without any consequences. In fact, as long as my joints function normally because of the cleansing of my system, I no longer strongly react, as I did at the beginning of the diet, when I occasionally eat a prohibited item. My worst enemies are dairy products: milk, cream, yogurt, and ice cream. In the summer of 2009, I felt pain twelve hours after eating only one big cone of soft ice cream. Was this due to the milk powder it contained? Probably, as some scientific studies have shown that milk powder contains high levels of glycotoxins (see chapter 4, section 7).

To conclude, the sacrifices that I must make because of the hypotoxic diet are nothing compared to the benefits I enjoy. In addition to the disappearance of the acute suffering that stole a major part of my joy of living, I have recovered the normal use of my hands and also a certain autonomy that I was beginning to lose. In addition, I have recovered the normal use of my knees. I can walk around without pain and participate in my favorite sports—like alpine skiing—with full pleasure. Finally, the long episodes of incapacitating acute inflammation that affected my spine after any light effort or any stumble while walking are a thing of the past. It still happens that I feel pain in my spine after I have been imprudent, but it is no longer an incapacitating pain and generally disappears within twenty-four to forty-eight hours.

6

MAINTAINING A PROPER PHYSIOLOGICAL BALANCE: PRODUCTS, PRINCIPLES AND INFORMATION

1. SOY AND HUMAN HEALTH

The consumption of soy is highly controversial. A close look at scientific studies on soy and human health is discouraging, to say the least, as these studies provide contradictory results. A number focus on soy isoflavones, mainly genistein and daidzein, which are molecules associated with the female hormone estrogen. Some studies suggest that isoflavones, or soy in general, are effective in the treatment of menopausal symptoms, inflammation, breast cancer, prostate cancer, heart diseases and osteoporosis.[1] Other studies mitigate these results. Such is the case with the meta-analysis by B.J. Trock and his collaborators on eighteen epidemiological research projects.[2] A statistical analysis of these eighteen projects suggests that a high consumption of soy can only modestly reduce the risk of premenopausal breast cancer. Another controversy stems from the fact that many women take isoflavone supplements to calm menopausal symptoms, but the efficiency of these supplements seems to be doubtful. In fact, a detailed analysis of a compilation of the results of seventeen studies on the treatment of hot flashes with soy isoflavones docs not show a significant reduction of this common menopausal symptom.[3]

Most of the concern about and appeals for prudence in soy consumption are based on data from experiments that claim that harmful effects of estrogen can be provoked by soy isoflavones. Some studies in rodents show that the isoflavone genistein can stimulate the growth of tumor cells,[4] while other studies contradict these results. There are also debates about the effects of phytoestrogens in children, particularly in newborns fed exclusively with soy milk.[5] It has been shown that the concentration of the two main phytoestrogens in soy is 500 times higher in urine and 274 times higher in the blood of soy-fed babies under one year old, compared to babies fed cow's milk.[6] Since it is not yet known whether phytoestrogens are biologically active in newborns, it's better to be prudent.

Toxicity studies that aim at verifying the possible negative effects of soy phytoestrogens on reproductive organs, particularly in males, also provide contradictory results. Many studies have shown harmful effccts in animals,[7] while others did not show any negative effects.[8] The main negative effects related to the inhibition of Leydig cells—cells that are specialized in the secretion of testosterone—is a reduction in the levels of testosterone in the blood, the number of spermatozoids and erectile functions, as well as the promotion of testicular cell necrosis. K.D. Hancock et al. established that genistein reduces the synthesis of steroid hormones secreted by the adrenal glands, Leydig cells and ovarian cells.[9] Studies on genistein toxicity in fish embryos have shown that this phytoestrogen has teratogenic effects that include embryo deformation.[10] Consequently, the study's authors fear that soy intake in pregnant women might affect embryo development. It would be beneficial to have studies that establish safety guidelines regarding soy consumption in different segments of the population.

Soy is consumed in Japan in the form of traditional products fermented with the aid of probiotics (such as miso and natto), and it seems that this practice is particularly beneficial to both the metabolism and the immune system. According to some, the intake of these products might be contributing to the proverbial Japanese longevity.

Another concern regarding the intake of soy is the secretion of thyroid hormone. Isoflavones can inhibit the activity of the thyroperoxidase enzyme, and as a consequence, inhibit the formation of thyroid hormone. A shortage of thyroid hormone can lead to the development of goitre and hypothyroidism, especially in individuals with an iodine deficiency.[11] A study carried out by R. Hampl et al. demonstrated that the daily consumption of 2 grams of soy per kilogram of weight affects the levels of thyroid hormone in healthy individuals when these levels are correlated with the quantity of phytoestrogen consumed.[12] Meanwhile, a meta-analysis shows that in thirteen out of fourteen research projects, there is little evidence that the consumption of soy disrupts thyroid functions in any way in healthy individuals with no thyroid problems. However, according to this study, adults who suffer hypothyroidism should avoid soy products.[13]

2. MINERAL WATERS

Most people who drink mineral waters don't think about the concentration of the different minerals that they contain. Some people like mineral water because they feel that it eases digestion. Others drink it because of the calcium it contains and which can have beneficial effects on their bone metabolism.[14] It has been shown that mineral water rich in calcium can, in fact, replace milk products, because its calcium bioavailability is equal to or higher than that of milk products.[15]

Not all mineral waters contain the same minerals, nor do they contain the same quantities of the various minerals. Studies have shown that a daily consumption of alkaline mineral water rich in calcium and bicarbonates and low in sulfates (SO_4) has great health benefits. Alkaline mineral waters compensate for the excess acidity of the Western diet and therefore reduce the calcium loss that results from such a diet.[16] Mineral water with a high concentration of calcium and bicarbonate as well as a low concentration of sulfate (mineral acid) has health benefits for the mineralization of bones.[17] One hundred fifty different types of mineral water were analyzed in this study.[18] Of these, 70 percent were alkaline and 13 percent were acidic; only 12 percent possessed characteristics that might result in a reduction of bone-resorption markers, specifically a bicarbonate concentration of at least 700 milligrams per liter (mg/l), a calcium concentration of at least 200 mg/l and a low concentration of sulfate. Mineral waters that are rich in calcium and bicarbonate are always relatively low on sodium.[19] The consumption of mineral water with the three above-mentioned characteristics was shown as able to cause a reduction in bone resorption not only in menopausal women[20] but also in younger women.[21] An increase in urine pH, which correlates with a reduction in acidic levels in body fluids, reduces bone resorption and significantly reduces both the quantity of parathyroid hormones and bone resorption markers in serum.[22]

3. BALANCE BETWEEN ALKALINITY AND ACIDITY IN BODY FLUIDS

Dr. Seignalet insists on one of Dr. Catherine Kousmine's[23] key theories: how necessary it is to good health to maintain the pH levels of bodily fluids (such as urine and saliva) at between 7.0 and 7.4. The normal pH of our cells and blood is 7.4, which is slightly alkaline. If we ingest too much acidic food, the excess acidic ions (H^+)

in body fluids have to be neutralized by buffer substances such as bicarbonate (HCO_3^-), albumin (soluble protein produced by the liver), hemoglobin and alkaline mineral salts such as calcium, magnesium and phosphorus to maintain the cell at a pH level of 7.4, which is a vital necessity. Chronic metabolic acidosis, or the fact that the pH of body fluids (including urine and saliva) remains acidic, has harmful effects on the body, including weakening of the bones. To reestablish the alkaline-acid balance, calcium, magnesium and phosphorus must be released into circulation to neutralize excess acidity, and as a consequence, bone mass is reduced.[24]

The ancestral-type diet consisted mostly of the consumption of vegetables rich in alkaline salts like potassium. Green leafy vegetables, dried legumes, raw vegetables, ripe fruits and almonds are considered alkalinizing. The modern diet has a predilection for acidifying foods: meats, fish, eggs, refined sugar, alcohol, tea, coffee, soft drinks, chocolate, legumes, refined oils, cereals and dairy products (with the exception of milk). Seignalet therefore advises that animal proteins be eaten only once per day to prevent excess acidity and that plenty of fruits and vegetables should be consumed. The consumption of mineral water rich in calcium and bicarbonates and low in sulfates also favors the maintenance of slightly alkaline body fluids and helps in maintaining bone density.[25]

4. PROBIOTICS

Dr. Seignalet recommends the consumption of lactic acid bacteria (probiotics), which are normal microorganisms of healthy intestines. The modern diet, based on the consumption of large quantities of meat, very often causes the formation of a flora of putrefaction. Probiotics counterbalance the modern diet by competing with pathogenic bacteria and promoting a more physiological flora of maceration.

Various scientific studies have shown that probiotics act by different mechanisms:[26]

1) They have benefits for both the development and the stability of microflora.
2) They inhibit pathogenic bacterial colonization of the intestines by competing with pathogenic bacteria and therefore preventing the bacteria from adhering to the intestinal walls.
3) They amplify the functions of the intestinal mucosa barrier by promoting the production of mucus and type IgA antibodies, which are specialized for working in mucus.
4) They regulate activities of the intestinal immune system, which is more intense in the elderly due to the weakening of their immune systems.
5) They prevent an overactivation of the immune system in cases of allergies or intestinal inflammatory diseases.

However, all yogurt and other fermented milk products on the market do not contain the same bacteria. Also, these bacteria can present different activity profiles, and their numbers as live bacteria may vary considerably. It's unfortunate that in Canada and the U.S., the government agencies responsible for food labeling do not submit these products to quality control to ensure that the nature and number of bacteria, as well as the supposed advantages conferred by these products, correspond to the declarations made by their manufacturers on their labels and packaging. In Europe, the European Food Safety Authority (EFSA) exercises a certain level of control over different food products. For example, in April 2010, Danone (France) announced that it was withdrawing its request for validation from EFSA, a request that would have authorized Danone to continue promoting, in various ads, the health benefits (and particularly the immune-system benefits) of its Activia (North America) and Actimel (Europe) yogurt. This announcement was made a few weeks before EFSA made a ruling on Danone's advertising claims.

Given that studies have shown that the information provided on the labels of probiotic yogurt does not reflect available information on the reduction of bacterial viability in yogurt over storage time, governmental control of these products is not uncalled for. A study published in British Columbia, Canada,[27] in 2004 analyzed ten randomly chosen probiotic products on the market, manufactured by different companies, and found that most of the labels do not clearly detail the nature and quantities of bacteria contained in these products. In fact, in two cases out of ten, there were no bacteria at all. When live bacteria were detected, their average number corresponded to only 10 percent of quantities declared by the manufacturer, and in most cases, the bacteria were also a different species from the one declared. Another study published in 2010[28] made it possible to evaluate, in a controlled manner, how long the probiotics lived—that is, the quantity of live microorganisms in yogurt drinks in relation to time. This university study evaluated the number of live bacteria in these yogurts after 1, 10, 20 and 30 days of refrigeration at 4°C (39°F) and found that there was a loss of 70 percent of live bacteria after 10 days, of 85 percent after 20 days and 99 percent after 30 days.

Also, since probiotics are sensitive to stomach acidity and are only useful to the intestine when they are alive, for best results they should be ingested in the form of enteric coated capsules designed to dissolve in the intestines, or that a number greater than 1 billion live bacteria be put into these yogurts. Certain therapeutic yogurts contain 10 billion to 50 billion bacteria per portion. When taken before meals, they seem to better resist stomach acidity. The Bio-K+ company in Laval, Quebec, Canada, produced a probiotic, Bio-K+, that has been the object of controlled studies on the prevention of diarrhea associated with the intake of antibiotics.[29] The last study, published in 2010,[30] showed that compared to a controlled group, Bio-K+, administered in the form of enteric coated capsules corresponding to a daily intake of 100 billion bacteria, was well tolerated in the elderly and reduced the risk of developing a *Clostridium difficile* infection by 62 percent to 68 percent in hospitalized patients treated with antibiotics. Lactic acid–fermenting bacteria contained in Bio-K+, *Lactobacillus acidophilus* CL1285 and *Lactobacillus casei* LBC80R, are therefore efficient in reducing the risk of diarrhea, even diarrhea associated with *Clostridium difficile* following treatment with antibiotics. This was a double-blind study that involved more than 195 hospitalized patients on antibiotics, between ages 50 and 70. This study therefore showed that this product helped reestablish a normal intestinal flora. Bio-K+ capsules are offered without prescription at pharmacies and in health-product stores. This product should be kept refrigerated in order to preserve the lifespan of the probiotics. It is also easy to make one's own yogurt at home, which would make it possible to consume it soon after making it and therefore enjoy the maximum benefits of live probiotics.

5. REDUCTION OF MICRONUTRIENTS (VITAMINS, MINERAL SALTS AND TRACE ELEMENTS) IN FOODS CULTIVATED DURING THE LAST SEVEN DECADES

It seems that industrial agriculture has led to a reduction in the quantities of vitamins, mineral salts and oligo elements in our food. This has been shown in McCance and Widdowson's work, summarized by D. Thomas[31] and A.N. Mayer.[32] Comparisons done between the 1940s and the 1980s on the quantities of the minerals sodium (Na), potassium (K), calcium (Ca), magnesium (Mg), phosphorus (P), iron (Fe), copper (Cu) and zinc (Zn) in twenty fruits and twenty vegetables showed significant reductions in the levels of calcium, magnesium, copper and sodium in vegetables

and magnesium, iron, copper and potassium in fruits.[33] It is important to be precise that only the publications of McCance and
Widdowson provide detailed information about the quantities of
various nutrients in foods between 1940 and 2002. Six editions of
their book *The Chemical Composition of Foods* (first edition 1940;
sixth edition 2002) were first published under the auspices of the
Medical Research Council and later under the auspices of the
Ministry of Agriculture, Fisheries and Food, Food Standard
Agency and the Royal Society of Chemistry. According to these
studies, it seems that for about seventy years now, there have been
fundamental changes in the quality of cultivated foods. Cultivation
methods, preparation methods and marketing methods have
caused a significant reduction in the quantities of micronutrients
and trace elements in our food.

The revised edition of McCance and Widdowson's book on the
loss of minerals in foods between 1940 and 2002, reviewed and published in 2007 by Dr. David Thomas,[34] provides very pertinent
information on the topic. The analysis of seventy-two foods,
including vegetables, fruits, meat, cheeses and milk products,
showed that there was generally a loss of 34 percent of sodium,
15 percent of potassium, 19 percent of magnesium, 29 percent of
calcium, 37 percent of iron and 62 percent of copper.[35] The reduction in the amounts of nutrients in foods could be due to several
factors, including a reduction of microorganisms in the soil, caused
to a great extent by the use of chemical fertilizers that render the
micro-ecology of soils defective. When plants grow in symbiosis
with soil germs, the latter increase the transfer of essential nutrients
from the soil to the plants. Experimental research carried out by
Gardens for Research, Experiential Education and Nutrition in
Great Britain showed that improvement of soils based on this principle can substantially increase the quantities of calcium, magnesium,
iron, zinc and copper in vegetables such as potatoes and leeks—and
at levels much higher than those obtained in 1940.[36]

Other factors like sun deprivation (harvesting fruits and vegetables before they ripen), transportation across long distances, time spent in warehouses and methods used to maintain freshness also contribute to the reduction in the micronutrient content of foods. The general decline in the quality of modern foods also results from the use of pesticides, herbicides and fungicides, and from the fact that the food industry's main preoccupation is the production of foods that sell well and can be conserved for long periods. Industrial production of food results in foods rich in saturated fats, trans fats, refined sugars and sodium, and greatly transformed meats. Foods thus produced are often deficient in the vital micronutrients. Also, chemical additives, such as coloring and taste and preservation agents, have been added to foods. We therefore have populations who have lots of food available to them, but who are malnourished. Many scientific studies have shown that this poor-quality diet significantly contributes to the increase in diseases associated with an inappropriate diet, and there is a significant link between a micronutrient deficiency and a person's physical and mental health.

Food-industry regulation: A shy beginning

Given the behavior of the food industry in general, which solely seeks short-term profit, governments have to enforce laws to force it to produce high-quality foods. There has been some progress in this domain, such as the food-labeling requirements implemented in Canada in 2002. This regulation makes it possible for consumers to know the components of foods as well as the different quantities of these components. Another regulation limited the quantities of additives like artificial color, preservation substances, sugars, salts and trans fats. However, we still have a long way to go, because in general, these are mainly recommendations, not obligations. There is no doubt that there exists a vital link between what we eat and our health; and so consumers, by demanding high-quality foods, can force governments to require the food industry to produce high-quality foods. It is becoming more evident that diseases are generally linked to an individual's lifestyle and therefore can generally be avoided. The stress of modern life, physical inactivity, a diet based on industrial procedures and the overconsumption of medication contribute to weakening the body's resistance to disease.

Industrial food and its consequences

For about a hundred years now (and especially since the 1960s), there have been significant modifications to our eating habits and lifestyle resulting from the industrialization of food production in Western countries. These modifications, which occurred within a relatively very short period, placed a heavy burden on the adaptive capacities of our genetic characteristics—characteristics that we acquired through a long evolution. Westerners are increasingly predisposed to inflammatory, degenerative and neoplastic diseases. Different factors play an essential role in the development of modern diseases: annual consumption of 44 kilograms (100 pounds) of refined sugars per person, tenfold consumption of sodium and quadrupled consumption of saturated fats, coupled with reduced consumption of vegetables, vitamins, minerals and omega-3 compared to the diet of the preindustrial era. Another possible, albeit partial, explanation for the weakening of our defenses against inflammatory disease in Westernized countries could be our difficulty in maintaining a sufficiently protective indigenous intestinal flora due to our more rigorous hygienic practices (as compared to past eras).[37]

Essential micronutrients have to come from food, because the human body either cannot produce them or cannot produce them in sufficient quantities to meet a normal human body's metabolic needs. These include certain amino acids, fatty acids, vitamins and minerals.

Oligo elements or trace elements are essential to our health but must be taken in small quantities. Therefore, the daily intake of selenium must not exceed 200 micrograms (or 0.0000002 g). Comparatively, the daily intake of calcium should be about 1 gram. Selenium becomes toxic when absorbed in large quantities. About ninety minerals from the soil are essential.

6. VITAMIN AND MINERAL SUPPLEMENTS
Seignalet's opinion

Like many other nutritionists, Dr. Seignalet recommends taking vitamin and mineral supplements (magnesium, zinc, copper, manganese, silicium, selenium, cobalt, chrome and rubidium), even though he acknowledges that the best source of vitamins and minerals is the most varied and most organic diet possible. He recommends taking liposoluble vitamins A, D, E, K and hydrosoluble vitamins B1, B2, B5, B6, B12 and C. However, he indicates that an overdose of vitamins A and D should be avoided.

Synergy between the various constituents of a food

Even though nutrition specialists very often recommend the consumption of food supplements, one must realize that a food's different biological constituents work in synergy. The concept of food synergy means that it is important to vary the foods we eat and to select those that are rich in nutrients. Food synergy is founded on the idea that interrelations between the constituents of foods are essential.[38] Synergy depends on, among other things, the balance between the different constituents of a food item, the manner in which the constituents survive digestion and their degree of biological activity at the cellular level. Getting micronutrients from food should therefore be preferred over getting them from supplements for the following reasons:

1) Given its role as a buffer, food favors the absorption of micronutrients.
2) Micronutrients drawn from foods can have different effects from those produced with the help of technological procedures.
3) In general, health is determined by the diet as a whole.[39]

It's clear that there is synergy between the different constituents of a food. Therefore, the proliferation of cancerous cells cannot be inhibited by apple skin but can be inhibited by an apple extract that also contains the skin.[40] The consumption of tomatoes has a greater anti-cancerous effect on tissues of the human prostate compared to the consumption of the purified lycopene equivalent. (Lycopene is the active anti-prostate–cancer element in tomatoes.)[41] Peanuts, when their allergenic proteins are isolated from their other components, do not provoke an allergic or inflammatory response; meanwhile, whole peanuts can provoke an allergic reaction.[42]

Evidence for the efficacy of micronutrient supplementation

The micronutrient-supplement pharmaceutical industry is founded on the idea that micronutrient supplements have the same health effects as constituents of a food. Clinical trials on supplements have shown that several do not work as we thought they did and that some (vitamin A, vitamin E and beta-carotene) can have side effects in certain cases.[43] A report by a committee of experts from the U.S. National Institutes of Health (NIH) on the use of multivitamin/mineral supplements in the prevention of chronic disease can be summarized as follows: most studies do not present conclusive evidence that the intake of vitamin/mineral supplements is beneficial to health, whether these supplements are taken in isolation or in groups of two or three.[44] However, this committee classifies the intake of vitamin D and calcium in a separate category. It cites certain studies showing that the intake of calcium and vitamin D supplements would cause an increase in bone density and a drop in the number of fractures in menopausal women. The committee concludes its report by affirming that the level of safety and the quality of the multivitamins/minerals is inadequate, given that those who produce them are not obligated to report side effects and that the U.S. Food and Drug Administration (FDA) does not have the authority to regulate these products. According to this group of experts, current knowledge is generally too insufficient to either recommend or discourage the use of multivitamin/mineral supplements for the prevention of chronic diseases in the American population.

Vitamin D and calcium

The majority of the Canadian population lives in regions where for about four to five months a year, it is impossible to obtain enough vitamin D from type B^{274} ultraviolet sun rays. In addition, the typical Canadian diet provides about only 5 micrograms (200 IU) of vitamin D daily, which is insufficient to maintain a serum level of 25–hydroxyvitamin D of at least 100 nanomoles per liter (nmol/l), the quantity required for optimal benefits from vitamin D. Canadians are therefore at a high risk for vitamin D deficiency, as many studies have shown. In fact, 5 percent of Canadians aged six to seventy-nine suffer from serious vitamin D deficiency (≤ 25 nmol/l). The average serum content of vitamin D among Canadians is 66.9 nmol/l; meanwhile, only 10 percent of the population attain the optimal 100 nmol/l. Until recently, numerous controlled studies on the effects of vitamin D on health used doses of 400 IU/day. In many cases, when associated with the intake of calcium, these doses turned out to be insufficient in the fight against osteoporosis, myocardial infarction and mortality in menopausal women.[45] However, in individuals sixty-five years of age and older, the intake of 500 milligrams (mg) of calcium and 700 IU of vitamin D per day moderately reduced bone loss in the femoral neck, spine and total body over a period of three years, and reduced the incidence of non-vertebral fractures.[46] Another study involving senior women who received 1.2 grams of elementary calcium and 800 IU of vitamin D daily showed that the number of hip fractures reduced by 43 percent and that other non-vertebral fractures reduced by 32 percent in comparison to the placebo-controlled groups.[47] A meta-analysis encourages the use of vitamin D_3 at a daily concentration of 800 IU in senior women, which would significantly reduce the incidence of osteoporotic fractures compared to the placebo treatment.[48]

In general, several scientific studies confirm the need for the intake of vitamin D and calcium supplements when these nutrients aren't received in sufficient quantities through food. This news concerns seniors in particular for the following reasons: with age, physiological changes lead to a drop in the photosynthetic capacity of the skin, a drop in the kidney's capacity to convert 25-hydroxy-vitamin D (calcidiol) to its active form (calcitriol), and a reduced capacity of the intestines to react to the active form of vitamin D. The efficiency of vitamin D can also be reduced by the interference of certain medications like glucocorticoids or by obesity, which causes the sequestration of vitamin D in excess fat in the body. In about 33 percent of individuals aged fifty years old and above, the calcium contained in their diet is not well absorbed by the intestines.[49]

At optimal levels, calcium and vitamin D play a more essential role in the cell function of many biological organs and systems, for all the body's tissues possess vitamin D receptors.[50] An insufficient quantity of these two elements can lead to increased risk for diseases like osteoporosis, colorectal and breast cancers, inflammatory diseases of the intestines, type 1 and type 2 diabetes, metabolic syndrome, hypertension and cardiovascular diseases.[51] Also, women who daily ingest more than 400 IU of vitamin D would see their risk of developing rheumatoid arthritis[52] and arthrosis[53] reduce by 40 percent.

The importance of the role of the parathyroid hormone

The parathyroid hormone plays an essential role in maintaining normal concentrations of calcium and phosphate in the body. It is itself regulated by the levels of calcitriol, the active form of vitamin D, and by calcium contained in serum. A shortage of vitamin D is generally associated with a rise in parathyroid hormone. Vitamin D in sufficient serum concentrations seems to ensure an ideal concentration of serum parathyroid hormone, even when the intake of calcium is lower than 800 mg/day. Moreover, a high consumption of calcium (= 1200 mg/day) cannot maintain an ideal serum level of parathyroid hormone when the quantity of vitamin D taken is insufficient. A very high increase in serum parathyroid hormone would lead to an exaggeration in bone transformations (remodeling), which will lead to a loss of bone mass. A hypersecretion of the parathyroid hormone would therefore play a significant role in the pathogenesis of age-related bone loss.[54] It is known that serum parathyroid hormone is the principal systemic determinant of bone remodeling, a factor in fracture risk.[55] In Nordic countries, during winter, at least 700 to 800 IU of vitamin D would be necessary to ensure an adequate level of this vitamin. During other periods of the year, an intake of 500 IU of vitamin D should be sufficient.[56]

Vitamin A, C or E supplements?

Numerous scientific publications consider that in the absence of any conclusive proof, it is impossible to recommend the intake of vitamins A, C or E or antioxidant supplements to ensure protection against heart disease or cancer.[57] Nonetheless, preliminary results suggest that antioxidant supplements could prevent age-related macular degeneration (destruction of the spot of the retina that is most sensitive to light) and selenium could help prevent cancer.[58]

7. CAN CHONDROITIN SULFATE AND GLUCOSAMINE SULFATE REDUCE ARTHROSIS SYMPTOMS?

Chondroitin is a sulfated glycosaminoglycan associated with hyaluronic acid, used in the production of proteoglycans (combination of a protein and glucides). Chondroitin sulfate is a component of the cartilage matrix; it contributes to the hydration of cartilage and therefore to its flexibility and elasticity.[59] Numerous studies have been conducted to verify whether or not this substance is really likely to improve the clinical symptoms of arthrosis. Earlier studies had shown that chondroitin sulfate could be absorbed orally and then identified in synovial fluid and cartilage.[60] Studies on the efficacy of chondroitin sulfate in relieving arthrosis symptoms have provided contradictory results. Among others, one meta-analysis based on five meta-analyses with controls indicates that chondroitin sulfate shows a weak-to-moderate efficiency in the symptomatic treatment of arthrosis and that it has an excellent safety profile and is therefore not harmful to health.[61] Another meta-analysis was based on six studies involving 1,502 patients; two of these studies aimed at determining the effects of glucosamine sulfate, and the other four, the effects of chondroitin sulfate. This meta-analysis concluded that glucosamine sulfate was not more efficient than the control after the first year of treatment; meanwhile, after three years of treatment, it provided a weak or moderate protective effect for the knees (an analogous result was obtained after two years of treatment with chondroitin sulfate).[62] It was suggested that chondroitin sulfate preparations from various producers and animal sources (that is, pigs and cows) could differ greatly and presented different modes of action. Certain preparations of chondroitin sulfate could have benefits for individuals suffering from arthrosis: it could promote anabolic processes and reduce inflammation. Other preparations might produce no effects or produce side effects.[63]

For its part, glucosamine sulfate is an amino sugar that helps synthesize many macromolecules present in different tissues, including cartilage. As is the case with chondroitin, it seems that the different studies of this pharmaceutical product arrive at opposite conclusions.[64] However, it is acknowledged that taking 500 mg of glucosamine three times per day has no effects.[65] There are indications that taking 1,500 mg of glucosamine sulfate once a day might be more efficient than acetaminophen (Tylenol) in relieving the symptoms of arthrosis.[66] One reason for the differences between the various studies is the disparity of the active ingredients contained in the different commercial preparations.[67]

8. ESSENTIAL FATTY ACIDS, SATURATED FATS AND TRANS FATS

About 60 percent of the human brain is made up of fat. It has long been known that fatty acids, among other molecules, help maintain the integrity of the brain and its functions (capacities). Essential fatty acids are important to health, but they cannot be synthesized by the body. They must therefore come from foods. Omega-3 fatty acids ensure the development and proper functioning of the brain. Docosahexaenoic acid (DHA) is necessary for the proper functioning and maturation of the retina and the visual cortex, and for visual acuity and mental development. Also, essential fatty acids play a major role in the synthesis and functioning of neurotransmitters of the brain and of molecules of the immune system.[68]

Evolution of margarines

Basing his conclusions on data available during his era, Seignalet affirmed that margarines were as dangerous as industrial oils. From the 1960s, many more studies underlined the possible role of partially hydrogenated fats (the characteristic of margarine responsible for its semi-solid state) in the development of cardiovascular disease.[69] During that era, margarine and shortening contained a high percentage of trans fats (39 percent to 50 percent) and a low percentage of linolic acid (6 percent to 11 percent).[70] In 2003, the daily intake of trans fats by Americans was estimated at close to 7 grams per day (g/day) for men and 5 g/day for women. The FDA, the American government agency responsible for pharmacovigilance admitted that trans fats in foods could cause death by coronary disease in 500 to 1,000 Americans per year.[71] This awareness and changes in the law regarding the labeling of foods forced producers to modify their recipes in such a way that currently more than 60 percent of margarines no longer contain partially hydrogenated oils. (These have been replaced with good fats.) We must, however, be vigilant about closely reading the labels on the products that we buy to ensure that what is indicated on the package corresponds exactly to the list of ingredients.

Changes to Canadian food-labeling regulations

Since 2002, the Canadian Food Inspection Agency requires food manufacturers to indicate the quantity of trans fats contained in a given portion of a foodstuff. According to a study conducted in 2008 on margarines sold at metropolitan Toronto supermarkets, food-labeling regulations led to a reduction in the content of trans fats in certain margarines. The proportion of margarines containing less than 0.2 grams of trans fat per 10 grams of margarine went from 31 percent in 2002 to 69 percent in 2006.[72] However, close to a third of the margarines analyzed still contained too much trans-fatty acids to be considered low in trans fats according to the agency's norms. Also, only the most costly margarines seem to be low in trans fats—proof that if we had to rely solely on the goodwill of the food industry, we would have to wait a long time for positive changes, except in the most expensive products. According to the U.S. National Academy of Sciences, unlike other fatty acids, trans-fatty acids have no nutritional benefits and should be eliminated.

Tests verifying the conformity of food labels

An analysis of the amount of trans-fatty acids in different foods available at the supermarket was carried out in 2006 at Minneapolis–Saint Paul to try to verify that declarations on food labels correspond to the actual amounts of fatty acids in the food.[73] Included in this study were 24 cups of margarine, 5 pounds of butter, 25 boxes of cookies, 19 boxes of snack cakes, 17 bags of savory snacks, 18 sachets of crackers and 5 sachets of microwavable corn. A second analysis made use of the initial sachets of popcorn and 24 other sachets, because the first analysis revealed that some sachets had a very high trans fat content.

Results of the analyses show that the different foods generally conformed to the indications on their labels (see table 7). However, even though the majority of foods in each category were labeled as containing 0 g of trans fats, a few contained this type of fatty acid (with average amounts of about 0.52 g per portion in the case of margarine). Savory snacks did not contain trans fats, and popcorn contained between 1.5 g and 2.4 g per portion.[74]

TABLE 7: Proportion of food-product samples with a content of 0 g, 0.5 to 2.5 g and ≥ 3.0 g of trans fats per serving according to the labels

TRANS FAT PER SERVING	0 G		0.5-2.5 G		≥ 3.0 G	
PRODUCTS	NUMBER +/ ANALYZED NUMBER	%	NUMBER	%	NUMBER	%
Margarine	16/24	67	8	33	0	0
Butter	5/5	100	0	0	0	0
Cookies	19/25	76	6	24	0	0
Cakes	15/19	79	4	21	0	0
Chips	17/17	100	0	0	0	0
Crackers	12/18	57	5	28	1	5
Popcorn (initial sample)	2/5	40	1	20	2	40
Popcorn (2nd sample)	17/29	59	5	17	7	24

To summarize, the food industry has reduced the trans-fat content in certain foods. However, consumers must read food labels attentively, because within a given food type (such as margarine, for example) the quantity of trans fats and of total fats per portion may vary from one product to another. Therefore, the quantity of trans fats in nineteen brands of cookies could range from 0.3 g to 8.1 g per 100 g.[75] According to food experts and public health authorities, trans-fatty acids should make up less than 1 percent of the total fatty acid content of one's diet.[76] Hidden fats—those that have not been identified formally—are mainly derived from processed and restaurant meals.[77]

The effects of trans fats and saturated fats on health

Saturated fats and trans fats increase the levels of low-density lipoproteins in the blood, which is dangerous to the body. But since trans fats can also reduce high-density lipoproteins (HDL), or good cholesterols, they are considered more dangerous than saturated fats. The American Heart Association recommends that saturated fats be limited to less than 7 percent of total daily calories and trans fats to less than 1 percent. Given that there are small quantities of trans fats in meats such as beef and lamb and in fatty milk products, they cannot be completely excluded. However, we can considerably reduce the quantities of trans fats we consume by avoiding foods cooked with partially hydrogenated vegetable oils such as shortenings and margarines containing trans fats.

Foods containing good-quality fats must be a part of a healthy diet. Monounsaturated and polyunsaturated fats (usually designated by the abbreviation PUFA) contained in high-quality vegetable oils (cold pressed) are rich in omega-3 and omega-6. Vegetable oils like canola oil, olive oil, sunflower oil and nut oils, as well as fish oils are all excellent sources of unsaturated fats. The consumption of soft margarines of high quality, that is, those that contain about 50 percent of unsaturated fats—10 percent to 20 percent of omega-3, only 20 percent to 25 percent of saturated fats and less than 1 percent of trans fats[78]—should also be preferred. Researchers recommend avoiding palm oil and coconut oil, which contain 30 percent to 40 percent of saturated fats, while some recent studies are less categorical about it. The FDA defines trans-fatty acids as unsaturated fatty acids that contain one or more double isolated links in a trans position.[79] Trans-fatty acids cannot be found in their natural state in foods. A law in Denmark prohibits their presence in foods.

9. EFFECTS OF SUGARS, ESPECIALLY FRUCTOSE, ON HYPERTENSION, DIABETES TYPES 1 AND 2 AND KIDNEY FUNCTION

Fructose is a simple sugar that can be found in foods such as honey and fruit. However, in the Western world, the principal source of fructose used to come from the sucrose of cane sugar. Nowadays in North America, high-fructose corn syrup (HFCS) has replaced cane sugar in industrial foods. It contains 55 percent free fructose and 45 percent free glucose (sometimes 42 percent glucose and 3 percent residual sucrose).[80] HFCS is used in more than 40 percent of foods with added sugar, including soft drinks. Since the 1970s, the use of HFCS has caused an increase in the consumption of sugar-added foods because it is cheap and easily mixed in industrial foods (for example, fast foods). It is believe that the added sugar—particularly fructose— in foods is at least in part responsible for the increase in the number of overweight and obese persons and all the associated health issues, such as metabolic syndrome, which includes insulin resistance, diabetes, hypertension, heart diseases and chronic renal failure.

Unlike glucose, fructose intake causes biochemical reactions that stop protein synthesis and increase oxidative stress and inflammation.[81] Fructose is different from other sugars because it generates uric acid when metabolized by the body.[82] In addition, when fructose is consumed with glucose, as in HFCS, glucose increases fructose absorption, thus increasing fructose toxicity and danger.[83] Fructose metabolism by the kidneys is complex and leads to oxidative stress and inflammation. Fructose consumption can also lead to an increase in glycotoxins, which are very toxic to diabetics. Consumption of fructose is even worse than consumption of glucose because it causes overproduction of triglycerides.[84] Knowing the importance of glycotoxins in the development of chronic inflammatory diseases, it is not surprising that recent work shows fructose, because of its structure, causes ten times more glycotoxins than glucose.[85]

Even though many studies have focused on fructose as the cause of numerous health problems, not all sources are alike. Fresh fruits, because they are also rich in antioxidants, vitamin C, polyphenols, potassium and fiber, may counteract the effect of added fructose.[86] But it's open to question whether or not fruit juices with added fructose, either as HCFS or as concentrated apple juice, retain the protective effect of whole fresh fruits.

A recent study[87] was done to evaluate if reducing only fructose and not other sugars could improve: weight loss, blood pressure, lipid profile, blood glucose, insulin resistance and uric acid level. Obese subjects followed a diet containing less than 20 grams of added fructose daily, while another group of obese persons followed a diet with a moderate amount of fructose, between 50 grams and 70 grams daily, with that fructose coming only from fresh fruits. After six weeks, it was found that the moderate-diet group experienced about twice as much weight loss while consuming fresh fruits, compared with the severely restricted diet group consuming added fructose. These results show that when fructose is separated from fruits it is damaging to your health. Both diets improved blood pressure and reduced uric acid and total cholesterol. It is quite revealing that a severe restriction of fructose with a small amount of added pure fructose was less effective than the moderate restriction, which allowed fresh fruits containing more fructose. In conclusion, added fructose is so damaging that even if those suffering from obesity drastically reduce their consumption of it, the little they would still consume would still be too much to allow for an improvement in their health. This study shows that three times more fructose can be eaten safely only if it comes from fruits, and not added as free fructose. It also shows that added fructose has deleterious health effects, but that the high content of antioxidants and potassium in fruits as well as their fiber counterbalance these negative consequences. The possibility that fruits may be beneficial and healthy sources of fructose is supported by epidemiological studies. In these studies, added free fructose is associated with an increased risk of high blood pressure, while fresh fruit consumption reduces the risk.[88]

Fructose, uric acid and kidney disease

Fructose has the capacity to increase the levels of uric acid in the blood. Epidemiological studies show a close association between sugary drink intake and an increase in uric acid levels and high blood pressure in teens. For example, an intake of 60 grams of fructose, but not glucose, per twenty-four hours (comparable to two 12 oz. cans of soft drinks) caused an increase in blood pressure in healthy young adults. This effect was not observed when the same amount of glucose was taken.[89]

In similar studies, added fructose caused a significant increase in uric acid levels while a diet low in fructose reduced both uric acid and high blood pressure in obese adults. The possibility that fructose may cause chronic kidney disease is more and more probable because this sugar has the capacity to cause hypertension (high blood pressure) and diabetes. It is a known fact that prior to the onset of hypertension and kidney disease, uric acid levels are high in individuals, including the young, and this symptom occurs independently of other known risk factors, such as overweight and stress.[90] Metabolic syndrome is a significant risk factor for chronic kidney disease, which suggests that fructose may be a cause.[91] For instance, daily consumption of two or three fructose-containing soft drinks is associated with an increased risk of developing albuminuria (small proteins that pass through the kidney in the urine—a symptom of kidney dysfunction). When fructose is given to rats with already poor kidney function, it speeds up the progression of kidney disease. This acceleration leads to swelling of the kidney (renal hypertrophy), proteinuria (a worsening of albuminuria—the first sign of kidney failure), glomerulosclerosis and renal tubulointerstitial fibrosis (hardening of the kidney with scar tissue and loss of function).[92] These anomalies are not seen if the rats are fed high doses of glucose. There is increasing evidence that added fructose can lead to ill effects on your health, including increased blood pressure, metabolic syndrome, liver changes and kidney disease. To protect your kidneys, researchers suggest that in addition to protein restriction, sugar, especially fructose, consumption should be reduced.[93]

7

THE IMMUNE SYSTEM'S STRATEGIES IN CHRONIC INFLAMMATORY DISEASES

The general ideas about immunology presented in this chapter are based mainly on Seignalet's[1] book and reference books by W.E. Paul[2] and C.A. Janeway.[3]

1. INFLAMMATORY RESPONSES

Inflammation is a defense mechanism against invaders that usually—although not always—come from infection. Through the vascularization of tissues, inflammation allows the transfer of the liquid part of blood—plasma—through the small blood vessels, called capillaries, to the site of invasion. Plasma contains cells that are specialized in the defense of the body, mainly white blood cells, also referred to as leukocytes. White blood cells are made up of different cells that come from bone marrow. Cells derived from innate immunity (that is, from the first immune system developed during our evolution—a nonspecific defense system that recognizes patterns of bacteria and of affected tissues) include monocytes, macrophages, dentritic cells, mast cells and polymorphonuclear

leukocytes, among which are neutrophils, eosinophils and basophils (appendixes 4 and 5). Biochemical mediators, like the large
family of cytokines, are made up of a wide variety of messenger
molecules, mostly produced by cells of the immune system.
Cytokines have particular characteristics and act on cells that possess receptors that are specific to them. Depending on their
specificities, cytokines can act on other cells if these cells possess
complementary receptors. Cytokines can act locally or even from
a distance in some cases.

At first, inflammation is a nonspecific response, because it
depends on the innate immune system; that is, it is directed against
any aggressive substance in the body. Unlike a specific immune
response, which increases in intensity once an invader is detected,
the innate immune response does not distinguish between the different types of invaders since it does not make use of any form of
memory. Because it is the first line of defense, cells of the innate
immune system play a crucial role in launching a fight and eliminating pathogens. The response to a particular antigen depends
primarily on recognition by the cell receptors of the innate immune
system of certain molecules (such as lipopolysaccharides) belonging
to different pathogens. Lipopolysaccharides are part of the structure
of bacterial membranes and are particularly effective in triggering
the innate immune system. If foreign substances are not eliminated
in a reasonably short time, the innate immune system and the specific or adaptive immune system collaborate to complete the task.

Unlike the innate immune system, the specific or adaptive
immune system produces very complex and variable receptors.
Although this makes specific recognition of an unlimited number of
foreign antigens possible, the specific immune system is more
advanced in terms of evolution and needs a lot more time to develop.
The specific immune system also enables the development of memory cells that have the capacity to trigger a fight and are a lot faster
in subsequent encounters against familiar foreign molecules or

pathogens. (A good example of a specific immune response is the response by memory cells that remain in the body after sensitization by a vaccine.) The specific or adaptive immune response is also responsible for phenomena such as allergies, autoimmunity and transplant rejection, which require the presence of memory cells. Because the specific immune system depends on memory, it is slower in launching a fight during the first encounter with a foreign antigen. However, it reacts in a more specific and efficient way to eliminate a known foreign agent. As such, when the specific immune system comes across an antigen that it recognizes, the immune response is faster since memory has already been acquired.

2. ACUTE INFLAMMATORY RESPONSE

By their very presence, substances considered foreign by the body send signals that cause an increase in the permeability and dilatation of small blood vessels (capillaries and venules). As a result, plasma and leukocytes such as polymorphonuclear leukocytes and monocytes/macrophages exit the surface of the blood vessels. Leukocytes go across the capillary walls and into tissue through diapedesis (appendix 5).

Drawn by identified foreign substances, these cells migrate towards these substances, secreting various mediators that activate acute inflammation while the cells ingest and destroy the foreign substance by an action called phagocytosis. This phenomenon is well illustrated by the redness and swelling that occurs at the site of a wound. Certain mediators are present in plasma; others are released by white blood cells during the inflammatory process; and still others are created by the influence of enzymes at the onset of inflammation. All these molecules quicken the inflammatory response. Pus is made up of dead white blood cells (cells that died in combat), dead or inactive invading molecules (viruses, bacteria, etc.) and cells from damaged tissues.

3. CHRONIC INFLAMMATORY RESPONSE

Inflammation is generally an innate immune response: a nonspe-cific response preceding the specific immune response. An innate immune response depends on polymorphonuclear neutrophils, monocytes/macrophages and a number of messenger molecules that are important agents in the elimination of foreign substances. Specific immune response depends on B and T lymphocytes and antigen-presenting cells (APC) made of up dendritic cells, B lym-phocytes and active macrophages as well as various messenger molecules, including a large variety of cytokines.

When the innate immune response has not been able to com-pletely eliminate pathogenic agents, an adaptive or specific immune response comes to its aid. If the adaptive immune response is also unable to get rid of the infectious or foreign agent, chronic inflamma-tion sets in. Chronic inflammation involves the immune system's principal or main agents, namely B and T lymphocytes in association with antigen-presenting cells. The most effective antigen-presenting cells are dendritic cells, B lymphocytes and (to a lesser degree) macrophages.

These different cells collaborate with the cells of the innate immune system and continue to activate the body's various immu-nity defenses by the secretion of messenger or activator molecules: cytokines. This results in chronic inflammation, which over time could lead to the development of chronic disease, accompanied by pain and the destruction of involved cells and tissues. However, the immune system actually launched the defense mechanism to protect the body.

Chronic inflammation can set in over many years in the form of subclinical (silent) inflammation, which remains below the pain threshold. This silence is what makes it so devastating. We have no awareness of its presence, even though it imperceptibly affects our health for years, and then comes the moment when we're diagnosed with a painful chronic disease.[4] The primary indicator of silent inflammation is the presence of c-reactive protein, which was discovered at the end of the 1990s and which is produced in the liver as a reaction to inflammation. Silent inflammation is the first sign that points to disequilibrium in the body. It is linked to hormonal changes that can lead to chronic diseases through the increased secretion of pre-inflammatory eicosanoids (very powerful chemical mediators that, along with other mediators, intervene locally in the inflammatory process). Hormonal changes also involve insulin secretions that cause resistance to the insulin and cortisol secreted by the adrenal glands.[5]

Chronic inflammatory responses and diet

Inflammatory responses, especially those that are chronic, are extremely complex and involve numerous molecules. In inflammatory responses linked to diet, the prostaglandins—mediators of inflammation—are of particular importance. Actually, depending on their nature and quantity, the polyunsaturated fatty acids we consume can cause an imbalance in the synthesis of prostagladins.[6] Excess type 2 prostaglandins derived from omega-6 and a shortage of type 1 prostaglandins derived from omega-3 will cause chronic inflammatory responses and, therefore, the onset and establishment of certain diseases, such as rheumatoid arthritis.[7]

Our diet also has an influence on free radicals. Free radicals are important because they are very aggressive oxidizing agents that can either have positive effects—the destruction of bacteria—or negative effects, if there are too many of them. In the latter case, free radicals can attack constituents of the body, such as certain enzymes, antibodies and elements of connective tissue. Our body protects us from free radicals partly with the help of protective endogenous factors that it produces naturally. Our diet can also introduce substances that counter the production of free radicals in our body. Protective foods are primarily those plants that supply us with vitamin E, vitamin C, beta-carotene, lycopene, flavonoids, thiols and certain minerals (Fe, Zn, Cu, Se, Mn).[8]

The production of free radicals is a normal physiological phenomenon. What is considered dangerous is the excessive accumulation of free radicals, often referred to as oxidative stress. Oxidative stress plays a major role in the development of the three pathologies Seignalet considers responsible for chronic inflammatory diseases: autoimmune disease, diseases of deposits and diseases of elimination/excretion. Oxidative stress can result from the body's penetration by foreign molecules such as carbon tetrachloride, ethanol, phenols, nitrates, ozone and insecticides. An unbalanced diet can also cause deficits in vitamins, flavonoids and certain minerals.

4. TOLERANCE AND AUTOIMMUNITY

For the body to function normally, its lymphocytes must tolerate normal cells and eliminate altered cells and aggressors. Antigens fall into three categories:

1) *Self-antigens:* These antigens are part of the self; in fact, they are the self. For example, all the self-antigens of an individual are called autoantigens because they belong to that individual and do not trigger an immune response.
2) *Altered self-antigens:* These are abnormal antigens found, for example, in an individual's cancerous cells. In such a case, they are called tumor antigens.
3) *Nonself antigens:* These are antigens that do not belong to an individual. They are called alloantigens when they belong to another individual of the same species; and are called heteroantigens when they belong to an individual of a different species or are from the environment (such as from drugs or food).

An essential element in our body's recognition of the self and the nonself is the presence in our cells of marker molecules called HLA (human leukocyte antigen). In fact, use of the term "leukocyte" is inappropriate in this case. This term was retained because the researchers who discovered the HLA molecules incorrectly thought that these molecules were only present in leukocytes or white blood cells. HLA molecules are glycoproteins found in the external membrane of cells and are part of the major-histocompatibility-complex (MHC) gene family, which are genes specialized in the recognition of the self and nonself. This molecular signature informs the immune system, in much the same way passports work, that an antigen or a cell must be eliminated because it is not part of the self, and that another antigen or cell must not be attacked, because it is part of the self. When a cell is infested by a virus or modified by a cancer, immune system cells will use different strategies to destroy any cells or antigens recognized as foreign as these are brought up to the cell surface via their association with the HLA antigens of the individual. If we did not have HLA antigens, we would not be able to maintain our corporal integrity. Any foreign cell could be grafted onto our body, and we would not be able to exist as a distinct species. This principle applies to every living species: each has a distinct method of keeping its integrity. Except for red blood cells, all the cells of an individual carry HLA class I markers, whereas HLA class II markers are present only on cells that present antigens to specific cells of the immune system. Cells formally recognized as antigen-presenting cells (APC) are dendritic cells, macrophages and B lymphocytes. HLA molecules are determined by genes that we have inherited from our parents. Consequently, each child is both similar to and different from each of his or her parents at the level of the HLA molecules, and as such, individuals are different from one another, except for identical twins.

5. THE ROLE OF HLA MOLECULES IN
THE IMMUNE RESPONSE

As mentioned above, the role of HLA molecules is similar to that of a passport. The role of HLA class I molecules is essentially to link to endogenous peptides fabricated inside the cells and to expose them on the surface of the cells.

So, endogenous peptides will be exposed on the cell surface in the form of HLA-I linked to this endogenous peptide that I call HLA-I-peptide-x. If the HLA-I-peptide-x is recognized by the immune system as part of the self, there is no immune-system reaction. If, however, peptide x is recognized by the immune system as a foreign antigen, the immune system will deploy its military arsenal to destroy the cell that produced the peptide. The phenomenon occurs when a cell carries a parasite in the form of a virus or an intracellular bacteria, or when a tumoral or abnormal cell is present. So, when in good health, an individual's immune system will effectively fight any of his or her own cells that have been transformed or parasitized by a pathogen once it discovers the presence of nonself molecules linked to HLA-I molecules on the surface of those cells (appendix 6).

HLA class II molecules are present on the surface of APC cells whose function is to engulf, digest and present molecules or foreign microbe antigens from outside the body to T lymphocytes. APCs are represented by dendritic cells, macrophages and B lymphocytes. APCs associated with HLA class II molecules link up with exogenous peptides—molecules from outside the individual that are therefore nonself molecules. These peptides, which come from bacteria, foods, drugs, etc., must be antigenic to induce a defense reaction. The association "HLA-II-nonself peptide" will be expressed at the surface of APC cells. So the couple "HLA-II-nonself peptide," expressed on the surface of the antigen-presenting cell, will be presented to a T lymphocyte that has the appropriate receptor for the antigen. After this recognition, the T lymphocytes will be activated and will start to multiply. The activated T cells will trigger different types of responses: they could secrete cytokines that are message molecules able to trigger various types of immune responses; they could also incite B lymphocytes to produce antibodies against the presented antigen, or they could request the T lymphocytes to change into cytotoxic cells capable of triggering attacks that will kill the abnormal cells or lead to the development of memory T cells (appendix 3).

It is important to underline the variability or the polymorphism of HLA molecules. The HLA molecules of an individual are genetically determined by both parents and could be very different from the ones expressed by another individual of the same species. This polymorphism originates in part from the presence of multiple genetic (allele) characteristics for every gene responsible for the HLA molecule's expression. Consequently, just for HLA class I molecules, at least 210 different alleles have been identified in human beings. If all the various random combinations of different alleles that an individual inherits from his or her parents are considered, it is not surprising that different individuals could have significantly different responses to the same antigen.

6. AUTOIMMUNE DISEASES

An autoimmune disease is characterized by an aggressive immune response directed against an individual's own cells or some of its constituents. This response is likely to have an adverse effect on various tissues or organs or to trigger functional anomalies on these tissues or organs.

Dr. Seignalet considers as autoimmune every disease that leads to an immune response that cannot be explained by the presence of living microorganisms or tumor cells and that has adverse effects on certain cells or tissues or provokes dysfunction. According to Seignalet, autoimmune reactions have the following characteristics:

1) The infiltration of the target organ by lymphocytes
2) The existence of a link between the disease and some HLA genes
3) The abnormal expression of HLA molecules on the targeted organ's cells affected by the immune response
4) The observation of an effective medical response against the immune reaction when immune suppressants are administered

Some autoimmune responses affect some organs in a selective way, while others have multiple targets. There are also intermediary forms between these two possibilities.

We have established that there are strong connections between HLA molecules and autoimmune diseases. These connections are of two kinds: the linking of some types of HLA with some diseases, and exaggerated HLA expressions. A great majority of autoimmune diseases are associated with some specific types of HLA molecules. This implies that more of these HLA molecules are significantly found in patients suffering from autoimmune diseases in comparison to normal individuals. So, the HLA-DR15 antigen is detected in 98 percent of narcolepsy cases, while the antigen HLA-B$_{27}$ is detected in 90 percent of ankylosing spondylitis cases. Individuals can express the HLA-B$_{27}$ antigen on their cells without being sick, but they have 141 times more chance of having ankylosing spondylitis than someone with no HLA-B$_{27}$.

The exaggerated expression of class II HLA molecules could also mean that such molecules will appear in great quantities on cells that normally do not express such molecules. This phenomenon could be related to an excess secretion of cytokines in the medium. These cells thus become a target for the immune system, leading to their destruction, as is the case, for example, with thyroid cells, which are destroyed by autoimmune response in the course of Graves' disease. It is also the case with beta cells in the islets of Langerhans of the pancreas in juvenile (or type 1) diabetes.

Another example is in cases of rheumatoid arthritis, where the cells of the joint envelope (the synoviocytes and the cartilage cells called chondrocytes) are destroyed by autoimmune responses involving the HLA-DRB1 gene. These examples show the crucial importance of the connection between HLA molecules and the mechanism of autoimmune disease.

7. SOME EXAMPLES OF AUTOIMMUNE DISEASES LINKED TO DIFFERENT TYPES OF HLA

The prevalence of autoimmune diseases in the European population generally reaches 1 percent. Owing to recent technological advances in genotyping, researchers have linked genetic diseases to many autoimmune diseases. Since 2006, the number of identified autoimmune diseases linked to genetic risk factors expressed in the form of HLA molecules has gone from fifteen to sixty-eight.[9]

Here are some examples of autoimmune diseases linked to HLA markers providing a genetic predisposition to diseases: acute anterior uveitis with HLA-B$_{27}$; ankylosing spondylitis with HLA-B$_{27}$; asthma with HLA-DRB1, HLA-DQB1, and HLA-DPB1; autoimmune hepatitis with HLA-DRB1; Behcet's disease with HLA-B51; Crohn's disease with HLA-DRB1, Graves' disease with HLA-DRB1, Hashimoto's thyroiditis with HLA-A2; celiac disease with HLA-DQ2 or HLA-DQ8, inflammatory bowel disease with HLA-CCA-1; pigeon pulmonary disease with HLA-DR3, rheumatoid arthritis and type 1 diabetes mellitus with HLA-DRB1.[10]

8

RHEUMATOID ARTHRITIS
AND THE HYPOTOXIC DIET

Seignalet classifies the chronic inflammatory diseases that generally responded positively to his hypotoxic diet into three groups: 1) autoimmune diseases; 2) deposit pathologies; 3) elimination/excretion pathologies.

1. A TYPICAL AUTOIMMUNE DISEASE:
RHEUMATOID ARTHRITIS

In 1985, Dr. Seignalet used his hypotoxic diet to treat a rheumatoid arthritis patient for the first time. My book and Dr. Seignalet's book, *L'Alimentation ou la troisième médecine,* both highlight rheumatoid arthritis because Dr. Seignalet's hypotheses were designed to explain the development of this disease and are the basis of his hypotoxic diet, which aims at treating it. (However, his hypotheses and diet apply to other chronic inflammatory diseases as well.)

Characteristics of rheumatoid arthritis

Rheumatoid arthritis is a chronic autoimmune disease that affects the synovial membrane and the cartilage of diarthrodial joints (mobile joints that possess a capsule—such as the knees, for example). The cause of rheumatoid arthritis is not clear, but it is thought that it results from environmental factors (such as foods) and from random factors (such as stress) in the context of genetic predispositions. Rheumatoid arthritis affects about 1 percent of the general population in Western countries. It is less prevalent in Asian and African populations.[1] For every man who suffers from rheumatoid arthritis, there are four or five women suffering from it. It is age independent. In Canada, about 65.5 percent of those affected by the disease were affected before the age of 55, and 35.5 percent were affected after age 55.[2] Rheumatoid arthritis is associated with the HLA-DRB1 gene of the major histocompatibility complex (MHC) class II,[3] as well as with a second disease susceptibility gene, the PTPN22, which is not an HLA gene.[4]

Based on the presence or absence of rheumatoid factors (that is, auto-antibodies against the nonspecific portion [Fc] of the antibodies), patients affected with rheumatoid arthritis are currently divided into two subgroups.[5] However, the separation between these two groups is based more and more on the presence or absence of auto-antibodies (that is, antibodies that work against an individual's own antigens or tissues) directed against citrullinated proteins.[6] Citrullination is an inflammation-dependent process that can change the structure and function of proteins. Citrullinated inflammatory proteins are more specific than the rheumatoid factor and constitute the best diagnostic test at the onset of the disease. Moreover, antibodies against citrullinated proteins give additional information on prognostics of the disease, because their presence indicates an aggravating factor for joint destruction and the development of comorbidities such as cardio-vascular diseases and other non-joint-related conditions.[7]

At onset, rheumatoid arthritis is difficult to diagnose. Diagnostic signs are not observed until the disease is at an advanced stage. In general, these signs are as follows:

1) Articular and periarticular morning stiffness lasting more than an hour
2) Swelling of at least three joint groups
3) Bilateral pain upon pressure on metacarpophalangeal joints
4) Symmetrical arthritis
5) Presence of rheumatoid nodules
6) Presence of the rheumatoid factor
7) Characteristic radiological images of hands and wrists

At least four of these seven signs are required to diagnose rheumatoid arthritis. Signs 1, 2, 3 and 4 must be present for at least six weeks.[8] However, patients who present only two signs are not excluded.

Detection tests for some antibodies (anti-citrullinated peptides) that are often present from the first stages of the disease have been suggested as a diagnostic tool.[9] Using magnetic resonance tests (a more sensitive technique than classic radiography) to observe bone and cartilage erosions in hands and legs has also been proposed.

Joints lesions

During the evolution of the rheumatoid arthritis, the synovial membrane, which covers joint cavities and secretes synovial fluid (liquid that favors joint movements), becomes increasingly swollen and thick, with many cellular layers that gradually transform into inflammatory granular tissues called pannus. The numerous mediators secreted by the inflammatory cells invading the joint medium (particularly T lymphocytes, macrophages and neutrophils), by provoking the thickening of the synovial membrane, cause erosion in different joint tissues: first the joint capsule and the cartilage, then bones, ligaments and tendons.

Forms of progressive rheumatoid arthritis that have no total remission exist, as do intermittent forms with pushes and remissions. Given the fact that the cause of rheumatoid arthritis is unknown, there is no cause-related treatment for it. Medications administered generally aim at reducing immunity and inflammation. They sometimes provide short-term relief, but neither heal nor hinder the progression of the disease in the long run.[10]

The evolution of rheumatoid arthritis: Genetic and environmental factors

Rheumatoid arthritis is a complex genetic disease. Many genes and environmental factors, as well as random factors such as stress, combine to contribute to its development. Research studies on monozygotic twins (identical twins) and dizygotic twins (fraternal twins) have shown that genetic factors account for 50 percent of the overall rheumatoid arthritis syndrome; the rest depends on environmental and random factors. When an individual who is an identical twin (and therefore shares exactly all his or her genes with his or her twin) suffers rheumatoid arthritis, there is a 15 percent chance that the twin will contract the disease too. Since the rate of rheumatoid arthritis in the general population is 1 percent, a 15 percent probability rate among identical twins demonstrates the existence of a genetic predisposition to rheumatoid arthritis. However, given that the identical twin has a high chance of not contracting the disease, it's clear that there are environmental and random factors at play.[11]

Environmental factors as well as genetic factors such as the HLA-DRB1 gene and the non-HLA gene (PTPN22) are therefore involved in the development of rheumatoid arthritis. The association of genetic, environmental and random factors can lead to the dysfunction of immunity cells and their secretion, which could result in chronic inflammation and the destruction of the affected joints. According to Dr. Seignalet, the immune response directed against joints could be provoked by a nonself peptide presented to T lymphocytes by HLA-DRB1 molecules that were abnormally introduced into joint-cartilage cells and synovial cells. Following this presentation to the T lymphocytes, the immune system activates. This nonself peptide, probably of bacterial origin, would likely be coming from the intestines, as the most probable way for environmental factors to penetrate the body is through the small intestine, due to its characteristics and its role in absorbing the products of digestion.

The role of food

Food could play a role in rheumatoid arthritis for a number of reasons:

1) Fasting sometimes improves rheumatoid arthritis, which becomes active again after the fast.

2) A gluten-free vegetarian diet is potentially beneficial to some patients suffering from rheumatoid arthritis, as it could cause the immune system to be less reactive towards antigens from foods that have been removed from the diet.[12]

3) A gluten-free vegetarian diet could induce a drop in low-density lipoproteins (bad cholesterol) as well as an increase in antiphosphorylcholine antibodies, which protect against atherosclerosis.

Dr. Seignalet's theory on the development of rheumatoid arthritis

• The modern diet makes the complete digestion of food difficult (as described in chapter 4 section 4). It promotes the proliferation of a perturbed intestinal flora that may contain a high population of pathogenic bacteria, of which *Proteus mirabilis* is a possible example. The spontaneous or provoked degradation of *Proteus mirabilis* or other bacteria by immune cells present in the intestinal environment can liberate the dangerous x peptide.

- There would be some harmful bacteria and the accumulation of some harmful foods in the small intestine in individuals in whom enzymes, mucins and defensins do not correctly function in the complete digestion of foods. This would lead to an attack on enterocytes and the tight junctions that unite them in the intestinal mucosa. The attacked intestinal mucosa could therefore become highly permeable.

- Because of the hyper-permeability of the small intestine, the x bacterial peptide would pass through the intestinal barrier at the tight junctions (appendix 1d). This bacterial peptide could have an affinity for synovial and cartilage cells; consequently, these proteins could accumulate preferentially in or around these cells. This accumulation phase could last for many years.

- We know that the initial outbreak as well as subsequent flare-ups of rheumatoid arthritis are often triggered by stress. These flare-ups could generate the release of a cytokine, in this case gamma interferon, close to the joints. Gamma interferon would cause HLA-DR molecules to appear on cells of the synovium and of the cartilage. These molecules would link up with the x peptide and carry it to the cell surface.

- The pairing formed by the HLA-DR gene and the x peptide implanted on the surface of the synovial and cartilage cells would then be recognized by T lymphocytes, which would trigger the immune response against the x peptide. This process would lead to the progressive destruction of the synovial and cartilage cells, which would in turn release substances that increase the inflammatory response.

- The inflammatory response would become chronic because the modern diet promotes the proliferation of the dangerous bacteria. These two factors together will continue to maintain the hyper-permeability of the small intestine. The permanent settling of rheumatoid arthritis could be promoted by the presence of numerous antigen-presenting cells capable of gathering the antigens released by the bacterial cell lysis—the destruction of the structure of the bacterial wall—and then presenting them to T lymphocytes. Antigenic stimulation would be maintained due to the continual arrival of x peptides from the small intestine. Moreover, the gamma interferon released by the activated T lymphocytes would maintain the expression of class II HLA on synovial and cartilage cells, which would make them continuous targets of the immune system.

- The synovial would be transformed into pannus (thickening of the synovial membrane) under the influence of released mediators by the cells of the immune system and by the sensitive nervous fibers. The extension of the pannus would lead to irreversible lesions of the cartilages, bones, articular capsule, ligaments and tendons.

Other variants of the Dr. Seignalet's pathogenic theory

When it is not a bacterial antigen that triggers an inflammatory reaction, an autoantigen (self-antigen) may be perceived as foreign by the body. Some T lymphocytes are intolerant of an individual's autoantigens. Normally these T lymphocytes are neutralized by the body; however, it could happen that some of them become reactivated by different mechanisms. The reactivation could be due to a cross-reaction from a superantigen (a highly reactive antigen that does not respect the usual specificity rules in immunology) or certain substances of bacterial origin.

The case of cross-reactions should also be considered: it is possible that bacterial peptides do not settle in the joints. The bacterial x peptide could induce an immune response against it after it penetrates the bloodstream. If there are any self-w peptides, which share a related peptide structure to the x peptide present in the joints, the immune reaction targeted towards the x peptide could also affect the self-w peptide. This means that a cross-reaction is responsible for the fact that a self-peptide or autoantigen could be attacked by one's own immune system. This phenomenon is called molecular mimicry.

The superantigen hypothesis

Many intestinal bacteria possess proteins called superantigens. A superantigen has an affinity both for parts of HLA molecules and for T-lymphocyte receptors, which have nothing to do with the specific attachment sites of this antigen. Consequently, since there is no very specific recognition, a very large number of T lymphocytes can be activated to trigger a massive immune response. This is very different from what normally happens when an APC-HLA presents an antigen to a T lymphocyte whose receptor is unique to this single antigen. In such a case, a small number of T lymphocytes are activated and are likely to trigger a normal and efficient immune response.

Seignalet's hypothesis and proposed action

In all cases, the causative agent will come from the small intestine. Whether it has to do with deposits in the joints of a bacterial peptide, a cross-immune reaction between an antigenic bacteria and a self-antigen located in the joints, or an immune reaction resulting from a bacterial superantigen or a substance from the wall of the bacteria, the intestinal imbalance phase always precedes the joint phase. According to Seignalet, at this stage, one must act as fast as possible.

Conventional medications intervene at a very late stage. Besides the fact that they do not target the cause of the disease, the different medications currently prescribed (such as anti-inflammatory drugs) target both the immune and inflammatory responses when the attack on the joints is already quite advanced. These medications are generally inefficient and have many side effects.

It is therefore logical to modify the diet. It is established that there are genetic factors that lead to rheumatoid arthritis and that environmental factors are necessary for disease expression. We cannot change the genetic factors, but we can act on some environmental factors—such as our diet, for example. Diet plays an important role in the process because the problem begins in the small intestine, where an excess of insufficiently digested food residue promotes the abnormal development of a bacterial flora of putrefaction. These two elements could attack the mucosa of the small intestine, which could become hyper-permeable, permitting abnormal quantities of peptides from poorly digested foods or from bacteria to pass through into the bloodstream, which is dangerous.

The hypotoxic diet and its results

The hypotoxic diet resembles the ancestral nutritional style as much as possible. It has six essential rules:

1) Eliminate all cereals except rice, buckwheat and sesame seeds.
2) Eliminate all animal milk and its derivatives.
3) Eat food raw as much as possible or cook foods at temperatures lower than 110°C (230°F).
4) If possible, chose organic foods closest to the original products.
5) Consume cold-pressed oils.

6) Take magnesium salts, trace elements and vitamins at physiological doses, as well as lactic bacterium.

The hypotoxic diet in practice: Seignalet's
treatment of rheumatoid arthritis patients

Of 325 rheumatoid arthritis patients, Dr. Seignalet retained 297
(34 men and 263 women) who followed the diet closely for at least a
year. Of these patients, 80 percent fit the American College of
Rheumatology's classification, and 20 percent met a more flexible
criteria, which corresponded to an early diagnosis. The average duration of their arthritis was nine years and three months. All the forms
of their rheumatoid arthritis were progressive, and partly or totally
intractable when treated conventionally. The severity of the disease
varied: moderate in 21 cases, average in 123 cases and severe in
153 cases. The average patient age was fifty-two years and one month.

Monitoring patients

All volunteers committed themselves to following the rules of the
diet for at least one year. Some of the subjects were treated only
with the diet; others continued with their medications. When
progress was favorable, Dr. Seignalet reduced the medication dos-
ages a little bit at a time until the patient was completely off
medication, except in the cases of failure. A report was filed at the
beginning of the diet, and others were added every three months.
Reports evaluated the characteristics of the illness: frequency and
intensity of arthritic attacks, number of painful swollen joints,
nocturnal pain on urination, number of times woken up at night,
duration of morning stiffness, sensitivity to pressure at the joints,
evaluation of physical abilities, use of medication and dosage,
erythrocyte sedimentation rate, erythrocyte count, and hemoglobin and neutrophil count. In successful cases, the diet was to be

continued for life to prevent the reoccurrence of arthritis. At the time of the evaluation described in Seignalet's book published in 2004, 20 patients had followed the diet for more than six years, 100 for more than five years, 126 for more than two years and 51 for more than a year.

Results of the hypotoxic diet designed for rheumatoid arthritis

Results provided by Dr. Seignalet for the remission of rheumatoid arthritis after following his diet were very encouraging, especially when compared to those obtained by conventional medicine. Out of a total of 297 patients, 56 subjects (19 percent) did not respond to the diet; 6 subjects (2 percent) responded partially in manifesting clinical improvement of close to 50 percent in their symptoms, but without any improvement in sedimentation rate; and 235 subjects (79 percent) responded positively to the diet. Of these 235, 104 patients showed an improvement in their symptoms of around 90 percent, and 131 patients showed a complete remission—a total disappearance of inflammatory arthritis, along with a normal sedimentation rate. In the group of 104 responders, arthritis was limited to small outbreaks involving a few joints, often caused by stress. Other clinical signs dropped remarkably. Their sedimentation rates, which were much lower in the past, remained above normal. In the group of those who presented total remission, those who had suffered rheumatoid arthritis for a long time and had significant deformities experienced only (but in a consistent manner) mechanical pain, the origin of which was linked to the destruction of bones, joints and tendons.

According to Dr. Seignalet, it is clear that this was not true healing, but a remission of the disease, since abandoning the diet resulted in a relapse in a given amount of time. Failure seemed more common among men: 44 percent, versus 15 percent in women.

Therefore, the rate of positive respondents among women is 85 percent. It should be noted that in 90 percent of the patients, benefits from the diet were noticed in the first three months. However, their sedimentation rates did not correct until several months after improvement in clinical signs. When a patient experiences benefits, the benefits last. Rheumatoid arthritis recurs if the patient abandons the diet and returns to his or her previous diet. In two of the patients followed by Dr. Seignalet, the benefits of the diet could be seen only after two years.

Dietary mechanism

According to Dr. Seignalet, the diet works in different ways:

1) By modification of the intestinal flora, in which there is a decrease of undesirable bacteria like *enterococci* and *proteus*
2) By correction of intestinal functions, owing to the consumption of foods that are better adapted to enzymes and mucus, which, in turn, facilitates the digestion of proteins, thereby leaving only a few thriving peptides
3) By modification of intestinal flora and the more complete digestion of proteins, which results in a restoration of the small intestine's walls that reduces the amount of peptides crossing the intestinal barrier
4) By restoration of oral tolerance—the body's development of tolerance towards antigens that have entered it via the oral pathway—after the restoration of the integrity of the intestinal walls, and thus a return to normal permeability

Under these conditions, the antigens no longer pass through the tight junctions of the enterocytes of the small intestine; instead, they are captured by the cells of the intestinal immune system, the reaction of which is adapted to the body's protection requirements.

2. REVIEW OF RECENT SCIENTIFIC LITERATURE ON THE ROLE OF GENETIC FACTORS AND THE ENVIRONMENT IN THE DEVELOPMENT AND PERSISTENCE OF RHEUMATOID ARTHRITIS
Genetic factors

As has already been discussed, the genes of the major histocompatibility complex class II named HLA-DRB1 represent the predominant determining genetic predisposition to rheumatoid arthritis. There also exist non-HLA-susceptible genes, like the PTPN22 gene in the population of European origin and the PADI4 gene in the Asian population.[13] In certain individuals, genes have also been identified that have a protective role in spite of the presence of the HLA-DRB1 genes.[14] The study of identical and nonidentical twins made it possible to demonstrate that the risk factors in disease development are also associated with environmental factors.[15] Environmental factors carried a lot of weight, since the rate of the disease among identical twins having exactly the same genes was only about 15 percent to 16 percent.

Potential environmental risk factors in the development of rheumatoid arthritis

THE INFLUENCE OF FEMALE HORMONES

Given the high rate of rheumatoid arthritis in women—two to five times higher than in men—it was assumed that female hormones play a part in the onset of the disease. However, the results of the studies on this matter were contradictory. A longitudinal study of a cohort of 121,700 women was conducted over a period of twenty-six years (from 1976 to 2002) to elucidate the risk factors linked to reproductive hormones. The study considered the variables of age, age at the onset of menstruation, age at birth of first child, history of breast feeding, use of oral contraception, irregular menstrual periods, body-mass index and smoking, with all these elements being integrated into a multivariate model of the risk of developing rheumatoid arthritis.[16] The study found that breast feeding for at least twelve months partially protected against the development of rheumatoid arthritis. Only irregular menstrual cycles and young age at the onset of menstruation were associated with the development of rheumatoid arthritis. Consequently, it is possible that the lower number of men who develop rheumatoid arthritis compared to women is explained by the protective effect of androgen (the male hormone).[17]

SMOKING (FORTY-ONE TO FIFTY PACKS OF CIGARETTES PER YEAR)

Smoking increases a person's chance of developing rheumatoid arthritis by a factor of 13 in both sexes.[18] In a study involving thirteen pairs of identical twins (monozygote) who differed from each other by having rheumatoid arthritis and/or by smoking, the smoker was the twin who suffered rheumatoid arthritis in twelve out of the thirteen pairs.[19] Finally, rheumatoid arthritis combined with smoking worsens the disease's prognosis.[20]

Many researchers hypothesized that in the development of rheumatoid arthritis, microbial agents could be at the root of the inflammatory process.[21] There is direct and indirect evidence that infectious agents constitute risk factors. It is possible that certain microorganisms trigger the onset of the disease.[22] The Epstein-Barr virus could be one of these microorganisms.[23] Many bacterial agents are viewed as possible etiologic agents in rheumatoid arthritis.[24] Several studies looked at the role of *Proteus mirabilis* and found evidence of a causal link between it and the development of rheumatoid arthritis. It was argued that there are molecular similarities in the genetic sequence of the *Proteus mirabilis* bacterium, like the hemolysine and urease enzymes, and certain human antigens like HLA-DR1/4 and the type 1 collagen; and that it would be equally true for certain peptides linked to susceptibility markers for rheumatoid arthritis.[25] Therefore, the cross-reactions between the microbial agents and the human agents that Dr. Seignalet hypothesizes could represent one of the pathologic mechanisms that cause rheumatoid arthritis.

The causal link between rheumatoid arthritis and diet: Not an "orphan" theory

Dr. Seignalet's theory on the role of food as a causative agent in the perpetuation of rheumatoid arthritis is far from being an "orphan" theory. It has been the focus of many scientific studies, and some of these studies confirm it. A majority of these works published during the 1980s and 1990s were the object of a meta-analysis[26] that highlighted the points below.

FASTING

Fasting appears to have anti-rheumatoid effects, as a rapid clinical improvement was noticed in some patients who fasted. An elementary diet would have caused an appreciable improvement of symptoms in some patients suffering from rheumatoid arthritis; the elementary diet involves consuming foods in their simple form: amino acids; mono-/disaccharides; and vitamin- and mineral-supplemented triglycerides. From a nutritional standpoint, the elementary diet is a complete diet and is also non-antigenic. Consuming omega-3 in its eicosapentaenoic (EPA) and docosahexaenoic (DHA) forms improves the clinical symptoms of rheumatoid arthritis in a non-negligible percentage of patients. The development of rheumatoid arthritis has often been associated with foods such as milk products, wheat, corn and beef, which suggests food intolerances as an exacerbating factor. In some rheumatoid arthritis patients, symptoms appear twenty-four to forty-eight hours after consuming the sensitizing foods and disappear after two or three days. Also, for the majority of rheumatoid arthritis patients, sensibility to certain foods is due to IGG antibodies rather than to IGE antibodies, with the latter being generally observed in allergic reactions. Food antigens in some patients cross the gastrointestinal barrier and circulate not only as food antigens, but also in the form of immune complexes recognized by the cells of the immune system or deposited in tissues. Abnormalities of the gastrointestinal mucosa allow the transfer of large quantities of large peptides into the bloodstream. Studies have suggested that rheumatoid arthritis patients presented abnormal digestive and absorption functions, probably a hyper-permeability to food antigens. Apparently, a great number of patients are seeing clinical improvements, such as the amelioration of joint symptoms, with diet changes.

Food's role in the development of rheumatoid arthritis

Following this scientific literature review and the conclusions that stemmed from it, the authors concluded that the possibility that food antigens can cause or perpetuate the symptoms of rheumatoid arthritis, at least in some patients, is high and is a potential point of interest.[27] According to these authors, the studies that associate diet with arthritis offer the possibility of discovering new therapeutic approaches that could provide a better understanding of the arthritis's pathogenesis. The authors end their discussion by underlining the necessity of differentiating between a healthy skepticism and the consideration of unconventional concepts in a bid to better understand and treat diseases.

Another, more recent meta-analysis also attempted to systematically evaluate diets or biological markers in relation to the development of rheumatoid arthritis.[28] At the end of this study, the authors concluded that it is evident that diet can play a role in the etiology of rheumatoid arthritis, but they observed that the studies were too few and involved too many variations in their design

to be able to draw definite conclusions. These limitations can probably be explained by the complexity of epidemiological studies on
nutrition. However, it seems clear that diets with a high consumption of olive oil, fish oil,[29] fruits, vegetables and beta-cryptoxanthine
(beta-carotene contained in oranges, mandarins and citrus fruits)
have a protective effect against a number of diseases, including
rheumatoid arthritis. The authors of the meta-analysis also report
that in three of the studies analyzed,[30] low levels of serum antioxidants are associated with increased risk of rheumatoid arthritis.

A major placebo-controlled double-blind study based on the
exclusion of certain foods was conducted on 53 patients with rheumatoid arthritis.[31] All participants had to undergo seven- to ten-day
periods of exclusion, during which they ate a limited variety of
mildly antigenic foods that they had rarely eaten in the past. Foods
from the individual's normal diet were then reintroduced one at a
time to determine which of them caused intolerance symptoms.
Each food that caused symptoms was identified and then avoided.
Of the 44 participants who completed the study, 75 percent felt better or a lot better after the exclusion of the foods for which they had
sensitivities. Objective measures confirmed these suppositions:
reduced pain and reduced number of painful joints, less time spent
overcoming morning stiffness, reduced time moving across twenty
yards, better grip strength, and many tests showing improvement in
levels of erythrocyte (red blood cell) sedimentation, levels of hemoglobin, fibrinogen and blood platelets. In this study, the main foods
that provoked intolerance reactions were corn (in 57 percent of the
44 participants), wheat (in 54 percent), bacon/pork (in 39 percent),
oranges (in 39 percent), milk (in 37 percent), oats (in 37 percent), rye
(in 34 percent), eggs (in 32 percent), beef (in 32 percent) and coffee
(in 32 percent). The other foods that showed an intolerance rate of
between 27 percent and 17 percent were malt, cheese, grape juice,
tomatoes, peanuts, cane sugar, butter, lamb, limes and soy.[32] This

study clearly shows that rheumatoid arthritis patients can benefit from the elimination of certain foods. It is also important to mention that the rate of blood glycotoxin (mainly due to high-temperature cooking of animal protein, whole wheat, French fries and chips) correlates with a certain number of inflammation markers in rheumatoid arthritis, such as serum levels of interleukine 6 and reactive C proteins.[33]

Two recent studies conducted among very different populations reported clinical benefits in rheumatoid arthritis patients who had adopted a Mediterranean-type diet.[34] The first study, from Sweden, reported in 2003, involved a Cretan Mediterranean diet. These experiments took place over three months on patients who had been suffering from active rheumatoid arthritis for at least[35] two years; twenty-six patients followed the Cretan Mediterranean diet,[36] while the twenty-three that served as the control group continued to eat normally. For the Cretan Mediterranean diet group, the main sources of fat were canola and olive oils, and the diet also involved the consumption of large quantities of vegetables, fruits and cereals, a small quantity of meat (consisting mostly of white meats), a relatively large quantity of fish (especially those rich in omega-3), little sugar and little fat besides the canola and olive oils mentioned above. This diet included only small quantities of low-fat milk products, mainly yogurt and cheeses (the Swedish generally consume large quantities of milk products). Results of the study indicated that contrary to those in the control group, patients who followed the Mediterranean diet saw notable improvement in inflammation, physical functioning and vitality.

It should be noted that the significant benefits obtained by those rheumatoid arthritis patients who followed the Mediterranean diet were observed only at the end of the three-month period. A subsequent study of the same group was conducted to examine the intake of fatty acids as well as the serum phospholipid fatty-acid profile during the diet intervention conducted in 2005.[37] Patients who had followed the Cretan diet and responded positively to it had consumed more omega-3 fatty acids and had a lower omega-6 ratio than those with no positive response. These data indicate that the individuals who responded better to the diet were also those who had observed the rules best. Differences in fatty-acid profiles were evaluated using three methods: a questionnaire, interviews on the history of the diet and analysis of serum fatty acids. The difference in the fatty acids profile can explain, at least partially, the clinical benefits shown in the 2003 study. Results of this study further confirm preceding studies that highlighted the role played by fatty acids in rheumatoid arthritis patients.

The second study regarding the effects of a Mediterranean-type diet on rheumatoid arthritis was conducted on 130 patients in Glasgow who had been affected by the disease for eight years.[38] After six months, the group following the diet had obtained significant benefits compared to the control group in the areas of pain intensity, morning stiffness and general health.

Dr. T. Colin Campbell, a world-famous nutritional researcher who has published more than 300 scientific articles, and directed the China Study,[39] one of the largest studies on the relationship between food and health, affirms that "the same nutrition that prevents disease in its early stages (before diagnosis) can also halt or reverse disease in its later stages (after diagnosis)." According to Dr. Campbell, "all autoimmune diseases involve an immune system that has revolted," and "one of the fundamental mechanisms for this self-destructive behavior is called molecular mimicry." Dr. Campbell agrees with Dr. Seignalet's fundamental idea, as he affirms that

> it so happens that the antigens that trick our bodies into attacking our own cells may be in food. During the process of digestion, for example, some proteins slip into our bloodstream from the

intestine without being fully broken down into their amino acid parts. The remnants of undigested proteins are treated as foreign invaders by our immune system, which sets about making molds to destroy them and sets into motion the self-destructive autoimmune process.[40]

According to Dr. Campbell, cow's milk is one of the foods that supply a lot of these foreign proteins that mimic our own body proteins.

9

OTHER AUTOIMMUNE DISEASES THAT RESPONDED POSITIVELY TO THE HYPOTOXIC DIET

1. ANKYLOSING SPONDYLITIS: HYPOTHESES AND RESULTS

Ankylosing spondylitis is a form of chronic inflammatory rheumatism that affects the lumbar facet joints as well as the sacroiliac joints (hip bones). With time, this disease can cause eventual fusion of the spine. Ankylosing spondylitis affects between 0.1 percent and 1.4 percent of the population. It is three times more common in men than in women, and symptoms generally begin between the ages of fifteen and thirty.[1] Since the HLA-B$_{27}$ antigen is present in about 90 percent to 95 percent of cases, and since in identical twins there is a 63 percent correlation in the incidence of the disease (compared to 24 percent in nonidentical twins), genetic predisposition to this disease is strong.[2] The fact that 37 percent of identical twins do not both develop the disease when one twin suffers it is also indicative of the importance of environmental factors in its development.

Dr. Seignalet's hypothesis

In general, Seignalet's theory on the pathogenesis of ankylosing spondylitis is based on the same principles as his theory regarding rheumatoid arthritis: causal factors are a modern diet that includes certain foods that induce the development of an abnormal intestinal flora causing small-intestine hyper-permeability, and the transfer across the intestinal mucosa of macromolecules from certain poorly digested foods as well as from bacterial molecules, both of which possibly settle in the joints. There could be a formation of HLA-B$_{27}$ complexes with some of these antigens, which would then be presented to cytotoxic T lymphocytes, and that would be harmful to joint cells. An immune response then follows in the form of the release of cytokines, triggering an inflammatory response that causes pain. In conclusion, dietary guidelines are the same as for rheumatoid arthritis.

Results

For the purposes of his study, Dr. Seignalet considered 122 ankylosing spondylitis patients who had rigorously followed his diet for at least one year. The average duration of ankylosing spondylitis was eleven years and two months. All forms of ankylosing spondylitis were progressive, and were partially or totally resistant to conventional treatments. Disease intensity was moderate in 8 cases, average in 84 cases and severe in 30. The average patient age was forty-six years and three months. One hundred six people were HLA-B$_{27}$ carriers, and 16 were not. A checkup was done every three months. One patient had been on the diet for more than nine years, 5 for more than eight years, 7 for more than seven years, 12 for more than six years, 7 for more than five years, 20 for more than four years, 23 for more than three years, 25 for more than two years and 22 for more than one year.

Out of the 122 patients, 116 (95.1 percent) responded positively to the diet. As with the six failures, the successes were unmistakable.

Seventy-six patients are in complete remission and no longer take any medication; meanwhile, 40 rate their improvement at above 90 percent and take only very weak doses of NSAIDs. Again, these are cases of remission and not healing: whenever the diet is stopped, there is a relapse of inflammatory rheumatism; and when the diet is restarted, remission follows.

2. MULTIPLE SCLEROSIS: HYPOTHESES AND RESULTS

Multiple sclerosis is an autoimmune disease affecting more than a million people around the world. It severely compromises motor and sensor functions caused by demyelination and loss of axons (the nerve-fiber process that generally conducts impulses away from the body of the nerve cell). Multiple sclerosis appears in genetically pre-disposed individuals; correlation in identical twins is 30 percent, and the environmental factors that trigger this disease are unknown. Genetic susceptibility manifests through numerous genes, with each gene having a moderate effect.[3]

Numerous studies indicate that there has been a marked increase in the number of cases of multiple sclerosis in Western countries (including Canada[4]) since the 1960s. More specifically, the prevalence of multiple sclerosis in Manitoba, Canada, rose from 32.6 patients per 100,000 inhabitants in 1984 to 226.7 in 2006. As this major increase in the number of patients cannot be explained by genetic modifications given the short time period, it seems evident that the rise in cases is due to environmental factors.

Dr. Seignalet's hypothesis

According to Seignalet, the primary environmental factor respon-sible for the onset of multiple sclerosis is a bacterium, probably *Pseudomonas*. This hypothesis might not be unfounded, given that in animals affected by experimental autoimmune encephalomyelitis (considered the animal equivalent of multiple sclerosis), high levels of antibodies against *Pseudonomas* and *Acinetobacter* bacteria as well as antibodies against white and gray brain matter can be identified.[5] A. Ebringer and his group suppose that *Pseudonomas* and *Acinetobacter* bacteria could play a role in triggering multiple sclerosis via a molecular mimicry mechanism.

The modern diet would be the second environmental factor. Seignalet bases this idea on the fact that multiple sclerosis is particularly rare in Arabs, Africans, Japanese and Chinese, but in individuals who immigrate to the West before age fifteen, it becomes as prevalent as it is in the rest of the Western population. The other factors are related to intestinal hyper-permeability: the crossing of the intestinal mucosa by harmful molecules from poorly digested foods as well as from bacteria, which is likely to trigger an immune response directed against myelin. Seignalet refers to Dr. Kousmine, who in twenty-six years treated approximately 500 multiple sclerosis patients. She reports that she followed up fifty-five cases for one year. She recorded a 97 percent unmistakable success rate in the thirty patients who rigorously followed her prescriptions.

Results

For multiple sclerosis patients, in addition to prescribing his ancestral diet, Dr. Seignalet also greatly reduced their consumption of animal fats and saturated fats and greatly increased their consumption of unsaturated vegetable fats by prescribing the intake of cold-pressed oils as well as fresh and dry fruits. He systematically added six capsules of evening primrose oil per day because of its richness in gamma-linolenic acid, essential for the synthesis of type 1 prostaglandins. In order to evaluate the results of his diet, he took into account forty-six patients who had been on the diet for at least two years, the longest having been on it for ten years. He recorded 1 case of failure, 4 cases of a slowly progressive halt in the disease's evolution, 8 cases of stabilization (including 1 case of relapse after five years of stabilization), 20 cases of net improvement and 13 cases of complete remission. A return to normal is possible only when the disease is at an early stage and the patient has not yet experienced permanent damage.

In conclusion, Seignalet's procedure in treating autoimmune diseases consists of 1) stopping the causative peptide (a bacterial peptide or food peptide) from crossing the intestinal barrier; and 2) following an ancestral-type diet that can restore complete digestion, a physiological bacterial flora and a tight mucosa to the small intestine. Because dangerous peptides no longer penetrate the bloodstream, the body can progressively purge those that had accumulated in the tissues. Seignalet underlines the fact that this method procures obvious improvement in about 85 percent of individuals with autoimmune pathologies, seemingly indicative of the fact that his method targets the cause of the disease.

10

SEIGNALET'S THEORY ON THE PHENOMENON OF TISSUE DEPOSITION AS THE CAUSE OF CERTAIN CHRONIC INFLAMMATORY DISEASES

1. THE DEPOSITION THEORY: THE ROLE OF INTESTINAL WASTES

According to Seignalet, all chronic inflammatory diseases have a link with certain modern foods that we are unable to effectively digest. These poorly digested foods induce a flora of putrefaction that promotes the growth of pathogenic bacteria, which attack the intestinal mucosa. This imbalance leads to the destruction or the disjunction of a certain number of enterocytes, resulting in the hyper-permeability of the small intestine. Insufficiently digested peptides of food or bacterial origin consequently cross the intestinal barrier into the bloodstream. Some of these molecules can provoke an immune response, and later on, an inflammatory response. This is particularly so with antigenic peptides and superantigenic proteins. These molecules tend to provoke an immune and inflammatory response, and then trigger autoimmune diseases. Other molecules do not have this immunological potential. These include certain lipids, carbohydrates, peptides that are too long or too short, bacterial DNA and Maillard molecules. These molecules circulate in the body and may be attracted to certain cells or tissues, depending on their structure.

The concept of deposition

According to Seignalet, when the amount of certain food or bacterial wastes surpasses the body's capacity to eliminate wastes through its excretory organs (the lungs, kidneys, liver, skin and mucosa, and intestines), these wastes then accumulate in either the host's extracellular environment or the cellular membrane, depending on their structure or affinity. They can even penetrate the cytoplasm and the cell nucleus. This buildup of harmful molecules has the following effects: a) the compromise of normal metabolic functions by the inhibition of enzymes; b) the blockage of certain nonenzymatic functions; c) the modification of gene structure and regulation; and d) the alteration of direct communication between cells due to receptor occupation.

Deposition causes modifications in cell functions, resulting in the suffering, transformation or death of the affected cells. The potential resistance of cells to this type of aggression depends on their capacity to eliminate wastes through the excretory organs and on the effectiveness of their genetically determined enzymes. We know that numerous enzymes are polymorphous and have different capacities. Since heredity determines the efficiency of human excretory organs, humans are unequal to the assault they face from pollutants from the small intestine. Deposition diseases are multifactorial diseases in which hereditary (genes), environmental (foods and bacteria) and random (stress, etc.) factors intervene.

After wastes are deposited in cells and tissues, various situations may arise:

1) Dysfunction of certain enzymes + little or no wastes = no disease
2) Excellent enzymes + lots of wastes = no disease
3) Dysfunction of certain enzymes + lots of wastes = disease

The outcome of cells subjected to pathology of deposition

Deposition is a progressive phenomenon and depends in great part on enzymes that are affected by this phenomenon. Each individual's inherited enzymatic baggage varies, depending on the type of cell in question (that is, liver, muscle, fibroblast, synovial, neuron cells, etc.), as well as the individual's capacity to continue functioning normally despite the accumulation of wastes. Generally, deposition pathology develops slowly. It is predominant in adults, especially in the elderly. It also worsens slowly. These characteristics distinguish it from autoimmune pathology, which usually affects young people, develops abruptly (at least clinically) and quickly reaches its threshold.

Cells on which wastes have been deposited evolve in different ways:

1) They may function insufficiently: osteoporosis, early type 2 diabetes, early Parkinson's disease.
2) They may function abnormally: hypercholesterolemia, arthrosis, gout.
3) They suffer: fibromyalgia, spasmophilia, endogenous nervous depression.
4) They die: Alzheimer's disease, final stage Parkinson's disease, final stage type 2 diabetes mellitus.
5) They become malignant: certain cases of leukemia, certain cancers (breast, prostate, colon/rectal, etc.).

The prevention and treatment of the pathology of deposition

Given that the primary cause of deposition (according to Seignalet) is the modern diet, a diet with no cereals or milk products and rich in raw foods and virgin oils, accompanied by magnesium, trace elements, vitamins and probiotics is recommended. As such, with the great reduction in the load of harmful molecules that these foods supply, the body would have the necessary excretory abilities to progressively get rid of accumulated wastes. When the various cells are thus ridden of deposits, this type of disease can be prevented, put into remission or even healed.

2. OSTEOARTHRITIS – A DISEASE RESULTING FROM DEPOSIT FORMATION IN TISSUES: CHARACTERISTICS AND PATHOGENESIS

According to Seignalet, osteoarthritis, commonly called arthrosis, is the most common pathology of deposit formation in rheumatology. Arthrosis is the most debilitating disease in the world. More than 10 percent of humans have symptoms of the disease,[1] and its incidence increases with age. After age sixty-five, about 80 percent of people present radiological evidence of the disease, even if in most cases, it is the disease's silent form.[2] Arthrosis with clinical symptoms is a serious problem both for the patient and for society, given that there are very few preventives or treatments for it in its early stage.[3] Current treatments try to reduce pain and improve joint function with the help of analgesics, nonsteroidal anti-inflammatory drugs (NSAIDs) and intra-articular injections of steroids or hyaluronic acid. These medical treatments have very little effect, if any at all, on the structural degradation of joint tissues; therefore, for lack of a better option, many patients resort to joint-replacement surgery to improve their quality of life.[4]

The most common symptoms of arthrosis are pain and the loss of mobility, which diminishes the quality of life. Arthrosis patients may experience pain from their condition only on one side of the body. The main joints affected are those of the thumb, the middle and distal joints of the fingers, the hips, the knees, the base of the big toe and the cervical (neck) and lumbar column. Contrary to other forms of arthritis, arthrosis does not affect any other parts of the body other than the joints. However, joints will have limited range of movement and can become progressively deformed (for example, Heberden's and Bouchard's nodes on the fingers).

Even if the pathogenesis of arthrosis is not fully known, it's evident that it's a slow, chronic disease leading to the progressive destruction of the joints. It was generally considered a cartilage disease accompanied by secondary changes that affected subchondral bone and synovial membrane. There was also much insistence on the wear-and-tear phenomenon as a cause of arthrosis. Even though wear and tear has a part to play in the development of the disease, *wear and tear is not its primary cause.* The old way of looking at the pathogenesis of arthrosis is now contested due to the discovery of abnormalities affecting the synovial membrane and subchondral bone at the onset of the disease. In fact, inflammation of the synovial membrane is part of the early events that influence the clinical stage of arthrosis. Immune cells from blood circulation, as well as other cells that line the synovial membrane, play an important role in the appearance and continuation of synovial inflammation by their synthesis of inflammation mediators.[5] These inflammation mediators, when released into synovial fluid, provoke alterations of subchondral bone, degradation of cartilage, fibrosis and formation of osteophytes.[6] Angiogenesis, characterized by the development of new blood vessels from old blood vessels, seems to contribute to these different phenomena.

Blood vessels of subchondral bone invade joint cartilage, facilitating the progression of arthrosis and forming osteophytes in the process.[7] Angiogenesis accompanying inflammation of the synovium can compromise the functions of the chondrocytes (cells that secrete cartilage) and the balanced functioning (homeostasis) of joint cartilage.[8] This imbalance may cause a redistribution of blood vessels far from the synovial surface, resulting in joint hypoxia (a reduction in oxygen supply), which greatly affects the proper functioning of cells and could cause their death.[9]

Seignalet's theory of the mechanism of arthrosis

Even though there has been marked progress in how much is known about the pathogenesis of arthrosis since the publication of the last edition of his book, Seignalet's hypothesis on the pathology of deposition, as an explanation for the pathogenesis of the disease, finds an additional justification in new studies conducted on glycotoxins. Seignalet reminds us that arthrosis begins with an alteration in the composition of cartilage, as demonstrated by analyses that underlined a reduction in the level of elastine, type 2 collagen and proteoglycans (complex protein chains linked to long polysaccharide chains) in the cartilage of arthrosis patients. Basing his idea on these data, Seignalet presents the hypothesis that deposit formation in chondrocytes could explain the abnormal composition of cartilage. He states that if an obstruction in the extracellular environment stops chondrocytes from receiving signals sent out by other cells, and if congestion of the intracellular environment disturbs the functions of their enzymes, chondrocytes become incapable of producing normal cartilage. They would then synthesize cartilage low in elastine, collagen and certain proteoglycans.

Globally, Seignalet's theory on the mechanism of arthrosis is based on the same theories as those for rheumatoid arthritis. At the beginning, the nonadaptation of our digestive enzymes to the modern diet leads to excess food macromolecules and, therefore, an excess of wastes and putrefaction that promotes the growth of pathogenic bacteria in the small intestine. Over time, changes in the intestinal flora activate the immune system, affecting the tight junctions of the intestinal wall, which become hyper-permeable. An abnormal quantity of food and bacterial macromolecules then pass into the bloodstream. Some of these macromolecules may have an affinity for joint tissues, which would lead to deposition pathology in the extracellular and intracellular environments, and then to a dysfunction of chondrocytes. These events may lead to the formation of cartilage that is poor in proteoglycans, eventually leading to its weakening, destruction and resorption. Basing his hypothesis on the fact that the problem started solely with cartilage (as had already been proven in his era), Seignalet placed subchondral bone reactions and synovial reactions at the very end of the process.

New scientific data confirming deposition as a cause of arthrosis and other chronic inflammatory diseases

Different researchers have established the presence of an angio-genesis at the level of the chondrocytes, which further reinforces Seignalet's hypothesis that deposit formation on chondrocytes hampers the normal functioning of these cells.[10] This angiogenesis could compromise the functions of chondrocytes and the homeo-stasis of joint cartilage. Angiogenesis problems observed in the joints could likely be caused by deposits in different types of cells within the joint. It's increasingly evident that the accumulation of glycotoxins, which are also called advanced glycation end-prod-ucts (AGE), is crucial to the development of age-associated inflammatory diseases. Glycotoxins are formed by the Maillard reaction, as mentioned in chapter 4, section 7. It is now evident that not only sugars but also lipids play a determinant role in the transformation of proteins and amino acids into glycotoxins in the presence of heat, and that genetic factors determine the amount of glycotoxins that will accumulate in various individuals.[11] The highest levels of glycotoxins in the body are found in the tissues that have the slowest replacement rates: tendons, the crystalline lens of the eye, bones, cartilage and skin.[12] Glycotoxins deactivate biologically activated proteins and enzymes by the formation of inter- and intra-molecular[13] crossed links. Glycotoxins affect the mechanical properties of the envelope and the renewal of various joint tissues, thus promoting the development of arthrosis.[14] There is a direct correlation between the intake of glycotoxins and glyco-toxin level in the blood in humans.[15] Therefore, the accumulation of glycotoxins highlights the primary molecular mechanism of those diseases whose incidence increases with age, as is the case with arthrosis.[16]

Results of the ancestral diet in arthrosis patients

Because there is a point of no return in arthrosis (that is, when the disease has led to serious deformity), it is possible that dietary prescriptions can arrive too late. Dr. Seignalet therefore excluded very advanced forms of the disease from his samples: for example, certain irrecoverable cases of coxarthrosis (joint degeneration with deformation and loss of the joint's ability to move without severe pain) requiring hip prosthesis.

One hundred eighteen patients, all suffering from obvious arthrosis affecting several joints, followed the ancestral diet. The results obtained were astonishing and unexpected, especially given that this disease is considered incurable: 99 patients (83.8 percent) experienced great and often spectacular benefits; and 12 patients (10 percent) experienced moderate benefits. Seven patients (6 percent) experienced failure.

The mechanism of nutritional change

According to Dr. Seignalet, it is probable that the halt in the flux of macromolecules from the intestines into the bloodstream, and therefore into tissues, stops the worsening of arthrosis. The fact that there is a significant improvement in the functionality of patients on the diet suggests that cleansed chondrocytes are able to resorb abnormal cartilage and replace it with normal cartilage— on condition, however, that there has been no bone destruction in the joint.

3. FIBROMYALGIA

Fibromyalgia is a chronic disease characterized by a syndrome of general pain affecting the musculo-skeletal system. It has numerous symptoms. On examination, there are multiple pain spots (varying between eleven and eighteen) on specific parts of the body; some patients clearly suffering from fibromyalgia do not necessarily feel pain at all these points.[17] Common disorders associated with fibromyalgia generally include chronic fatigue, sleep disorders and episodes of depression.[18] It is now known that these symptoms are not caused by peripheral or inflammatory damage, and there are suspicions that there may be fundamental problems in the body's ways of being sensitive to pain rather than an abnormality confined to the part of the body where the pain is felt.[19] In most countries, the disease's prevalence varies from 2 percent to 7 percent of the population, and is more prevalent in women and the elderly. Studies conducted on identical twins suggest that the risk of developing this disease is due 50 percent to genetic factors and 50 percent to environmental or random factors, such as stress.[20] Most conventional treatments and alternative medicine only provide moderate improvement in patients' symptoms and functional abilities.[21]

Fibromyalgia and the deposit phenomenon

Seignalet attributes the onset of fibromyalgia to progressive deposit accumulation of bacterial and food molecules from the small intestine onto muscle, tendon and brain cells. In fact, poorly digested bacterial and food molecules could cross into the bloodstream and be deposited in the muscles, tendons, neurons and astrocytes (the latter being the nourishing cells of the neurons). Deposit formation in these cells could cause a deregulation of normal functions, provoking pain in muscles and tendons as well as problems caused by the nervous system. As deposition increases slowly and gradually through the years, fibromyalgia does not generally manifest itself until one reaches one's adult years, and its development is a function of genetic predispositions and environmental factors.

Results obtained with the ancestral diet

Eighty fibromyalgia patients (72 women and 8 men) participated in Seignalet's study. Patients had been on the hypotoxic diet for between one and ten years. The diet caused a complete remission in 58 patients (72.5 percent) whose symptoms disappeared completely. Ten patients reported improvement of about 75 percent; four patients reported improvement of about 50 percent. There were eight cases of failure.

Positive effects were generally observed after a few weeks and would progressively increase within three months to two years. Whenever there was a departure from the diet, the less severe symptoms of fibromyalgia would resurface. For the disease to remain in a state of remission, patients had to remain on the diet.

4. TYPE 2 OR NON-INSULIN-DEPENDENT DIABETES

Obesity is currently a very serious health problem worldwide. Epidemiological studies indicate that overweight, obesity and lack of physical activity are major risk factors for type 2 diabetes.[22] More than 300 million people present a reduced glucose tolerance and 246 million people suffer from type 2 diabetes.[23] Cases of diabetes are constantly increasing: a 50 percent increase in the incidence of diabetes has been observed in the United States between 1973 and 1993.[24] Other studies conducted in different countries also report marked increases in the prevalence of type 2 diabetes in recent decades.[25] Since we know that type 2 diabetes is of both polygenic and environmental origin, we can assume that it is the lifestyle of the population and not the genes that have changed, given the short lapse of time.

Obesity is associated with the silent, or subclinical, inflammation of adipose tissue that may lead to chronic activation of the innate immune system, which could later lead to insulin resistance and to type 2 diabetes.[26] This situation is characterized by the secretion of numerous inflammatory molecules that have local and systemic effects on various organs. Insulin resistance can be defined as the inability of insulin, a hypoglycemic hormone, to carry out its normal functions, even though the beta cells of the pancreas continue to secrete it.[27] In 2005, the International Diabetes Federation established the following criteria for the clinical diagnosis of type 2 diabetes: visceral obesity, increased triglycerides, reduced HDL levels (high-density lipoproteins—good cholesterol), the presence of hypertension and reduced glucose tolerance.[28] Available medications can slow the evolution of the disease and delay the onset of complications, but they do not heal the disease and can have side effects.[29]

The pathogenesis of type 2 diabetes: Seignalet's hypothesis

Ill-adapted to our digestive enzymes, our modern diet can cause a modification of intestinal flora as well as the formation of excessive food and bacterial macromolecules in the small intestine. This situation may result in an attack on the mucosa of the small intestine and an excessive increase in its permeability. The transfer of macromolecules into the bloodstream could provoke deposition in the pancreatic beta cells, which secrete insulin, especially if the patient's excretory organs are genetically less efficient. Obesity and a sedentary lifestyle amplify the phenomenon of deposition of target insulin cells, thus causing a resistance to insulin and hyperglycemia. Diabetics produce an abnormally large amount of endogenous glycotoxins (that is, glycotoxins produced by the body itself). These glycotoxins link up with the RAGEs of all affected cells in atherosclerosis, provoking inflammatory reactions. The latter may alter vascular walls by inducing accelerated aging of the arteries and arterioles, which would cause vascular complications in type 2 diabetes.

Effects of the hypotoxic diet on the intestine

The goal of Seignalet's hypotoxic diet is to normalize the food and bacterial content of the small intestine and restore its tightness. Therefore, while the hypotoxic diet stops the migration of harmful molecules into the bloodstream, the body must be able to progressively purge the exogenous wastes of altered cells in individuals genetically predisposed to type 2 diabetes. According to Seignalet, it is essential to change the diet as early as possible, while there are still a sufficient number of beta cells to produce insulin.

Results

Twenty-five type 2 diabetes patients took part in this study. These patients were sixty-one years old on average, and had suffered diabetes for a duration ranging from one year to thirty-three years, with the average being twelve years. Their fasting blood sugar levels were between 1.40 grams and 3.50 grams per liter (g/liter), the normal levels being 1 g/liter. The glycosylated hemoglobin percentage was between 6.7 percent and 9.3 percent, depending on the patient. Eight patients had already suffered vascular complications. All the patients were on one or more medications for diabetes. None of the patients had reached the stage of insulin dependence.

The hypotoxic diet put the disease in remission for twenty patients, who stopped all medication. Benefits appeared after a few weeks. Success criteria included a fasting glycemia that was equal to or lower than 1 gram per liter and a glycosylated hemoglobin percentage equal to or lower than 6 percent. The patients had been on the diet for a period of between six months (patient with shortest diet duration) and six years (patient with longest diet duration). The five other patients saw a marked improvement in their state. Their levels of fasting glycemia had been brought back to a percentage ranging between 35 percent and 55 percent of their initial value and were between 1.2 grams and 1.7 grams. Their glycosylated hemoglobin levels went down to below 8 percent, reducing vascular risk. It is important to repeat the fact that these cases were remission—not healing—and that to continue to enjoy its benefits, patients must stay on the hypotoxic diet for life.

11

DISEASES OF ELIMINATION

1. SEIGNALET'S THEORY OF DISEASES OF ELIMINATION

Numerous molecules, such as certain molecules derived from the Maillard reaction, bacterial cell-wall lipopolysaccharides, carbohydrate isomers, lipids and proteins, cannot be degraded by human enzymes. Therefore, these molecules must be eliminated by the various excretory organs. The excretory organs are the kidneys, the liver, the intestines, the lungs, the skin and the mucus membranes. White blood cells play a primary role as waste collectors in this process of elimination.

When the harmful molecules to be eliminated are few, a physiological elimination takes place at the level of the excretory organs. Seignalet hypothesizes that physiological elimination is rarely observed in individuals eating a modern diet, because the cleansing processes are usually blocked. It is, however, clear that genetic factors have an influence on the efficacy of the excretory organs, and resistance to excesses and the capacity to eliminate wastes vary from one individual to another.

Pathological elimination occurs when harmful molecules are abundant, and as a result, activated white blood cells increase in number and provoke inflammation of the excretory organs by the secreting cytokines. In the long run, the continuous secretion of cytokines induces a chronic inflammation of the excretory organs, which can trigger different diseases depending on the affected excretory organ and the individual's genetic predisposition. For example, if the digestive tract is chronically inflamed, there may be an onset of colitis or Crohn's disease. If the skin is inflamed, there may be acne, certain eczemas and psoriasis; or infections could develop in the mucosal membranes of the ears, neck and throat, such as otitis, sinusitis or conjunctivitis.

To prevent diseases of elimination, Seignalet recommends the ancestral diet, which can greatly reduce the supply of dangerous molecules to the body and promote both their elimination and the cleansing of the excretory organs.

2. COLITIS OR IRRITABLE BOWEL SYNDROME

Inflammatory diseases of the intestines are multifactorial diseases. Their onset depends on both genetic predisposition and environmental triggers. Colitis, also called irritable bowel syndrome or functional colopathy, is very common in Western countries and is manifested by abdominal pain and bloating, as well as constipation, diarrhea or an alternation of both. According to Seignalet, its pathogenesis is due to the modern diet and therefore to the same mechanisms as those that cause other inflammatory diseases. The very early stages of colitis affect the small intestine; only much later is the colon affected.

Dr. Seignalet tested his hypotoxic diet on 237 patients with early colitis who also had no history of amebiasis (the presence of parasites called amebas). There was complete remission in 233 patients, generally after one month. All clinical signs progressively disappeared. Three people saw only a partial improvement, and in two cases, there was total failure.

3. CROHN'S DISEASE

Crohn's disease is characterized by an inflammation of the small intestine. It is a multifactorial disease in which hereditary, infections, environmental factors, the immune state of the host, intestinal flora, food allergies and hypersensitivity can play a role.[1] The importance of environmental factors is underlined by the fact that long-term studies show a general increase in the incidence of Crohn's during the twentieth century.[2] Recent studies demonstrate that intestinal hyper-permeability plays a critical role in the etiology of pediatric Crohn's disease.[3] Intestinal hyper-permeability favors the penetration of pathogens, toxic compositions and macromolecules into the bloodstream.

Here again, Dr. Seignalet's hypothesis on the pathogenesis of the disease is based on the modern diet and hyper-permeability of the intestine. A phenomenon that is much more inflammatory than immune may occur after macromolecules are captured by polymorphonuclear leukocytes and macrophages. Later, infiltrations of leukocytes and ulcerations may be observed in the epithelium of the terminal ileum with desquamation of epithelial cells (the loss of bits of mucosa by peeling or by excess shedding).

Dr. Seignalet put 99 Crohn's patients on the hypotoxic diet. Of these, he considered only 72 patients who had been on the hypotoxic diet for at least one year. He recorded 62 cases of total success (86 percent) with total or quasi-total remission, 9 cases of average results (12.5 percent) and only 1 case of total failure (1.4 percent).

4. ACNE: A SKIN PATHOLOGY
INVOLVING EXCRETION

More than 17 million Americans suffer from acne, and between 80 percent and 90 percent of adolescents are affected by this pathology to different degrees.[4] In general, acne results from the clogging and inflammation of hair follicles and their associated sebaceous glands. Acne may depend on an inflammatory phenomenon and imply the colonization of hair follicles by bacteria. Hormonal activity, production of sebum and clogging of follicles can make this phenomenon worse. Environmental factors like nutritional choices also play a role in the prevalence of acne. Numerous studies on a large number of adolescents and involving adequate control groups have shown that a diet rich in milk products is associated both with an increased risk of acne and with the severity of the disease.[5] Milk components such as the insulin-like growth factor 1 (IGF-1) play a role in acne's development.[6] Also, a high-glycemic-index diet may influence the duration of acne.[7] There are multiple treatment methods for acne, including medication for topical administration, anti-inflammatories, antibiotics, hormone therapy and phototherapy.[8] These treatments are usually disappointing.

Seignalet's hypothesis on the pathogenesis of acne, like the other pathologies that he successfully treated, is first of all based on the migration of partially degraded food and bacterial macromolecules into body tissues via the mucosa of the small intestine, which has become hyper-permeable. These molecules can be captured by polymorphonuclear neutrophils that may go all the way to the skin surrounding sebaceous glands. These neutrophils carry harmful molecules that secrete cytokines, which in turn may incite epithelial cells to multiply and glandular tissue to secrete sebum that is too plentiful and too thick. Clogging of the sebaceous glands can result and may sometimes provoke a bacterial superinfection and the formation of pustules.

Seignalet used his hypotoxic diet on 42 acne patients. Acne totally regressed in 40 patients, while in the 2 other patients, inflamed lesions clearly reduced. However, Seignalet stresses that scarring from previous outbreaks is irreversible—hence the importance of early treatment.

5. ATOPIC ECZEMA (ALSO CALLED ATOPIC DERMATITIS)

Atopic eczema is a chronic disease characterized by symptoms like itching. This disease affects about 17 percent of children in developed countries. The prevalence of eczema has been on the increase since the 1950s and 1960s in countries whose lifestyle resembles that of the West.[9] The cause of eczema is multifactorial: the interaction of genetics and the environment is an early factor in the pathogenesis of the disease.[10] Intestinal flora may be involved in the development of atopic eczema in young children.[11] Despite the importance of this disease from a public-health point of view, the efficacy of available treatments is insufficient. Corticosteroids are the most effective topical treatments, but these must be used only for a short time because of their side effects.[12]

According to Seignalet, eczema results from a disease of elimination based on phenomena similar to those described for acne, and that means the excretory organs are at risk. Dr. Seignalet tested his diet on 43 atopic eczema patients. Total success was recorded in 36 patients, a marked improvement in 4 patients and failure in 3 patients.

6. ASTHMA

Asthma is a chronic inflammatory disease of the respiratory system and is characterized by reversible obstruction of the respiratory tract, hyperreactivity, infiltration of white blood cells into the submucosa of the respiratory tract, hypersecretion of mucus and remodeling of the respiratory tract.[13] This disease involves the presence of an allergen and the modulation of an allergic response.[14]

Asthma is the most common chronic disease in children, and in 2007, more than 9.5 million American children were diagnosed with asthma (13 percent).[15] In Ontario, Canada, the prevalence of asthma in children under ten years of age went from 146.6 cases per 1,000 children between 1994 and 1995 to 196.2 cases per 1,000 children in 1998 to 1999, representing a 34.8 percent increase in approximately five years.[16] The prevalence of asthma has been constantly increasing for many decades now, as is the case with most chronic inflammatory diseases. Asthma is more than a poly-genetic disease affected by environmental factors.[17] The usual treatment of asthma is largely based on the use of anti-inflammatory corticosteroids and bronchodilators that do not cure the disease.[18]

Dr. Seignalet considers asthma first of all as an inflammatory disease that is also a disease of elimination. He formulates the following theory: macromolecules from the small intestine are transported by white blood cells to be eliminated by the bronchial walls. The excessive presence of different white blood cells at this point may liberate cytokines, which may cause an inflammatory infiltration of the bronchial submucosa. Wastes may then be expulsed in bronchial secretions and desquamations (the loss of epidermis cells). Chronic respiratory inflammation may increase in the presence of factors like allergens, pollutants, cold, exercise and stress.

In 2005, scientists showed that intestinal hyper-permeability could be involved in the pathogenesis of many pediatric chronic diseases due to the immaturity of the intestinal barrier in children with a genetic predisposition.[19] They stressed the importance of the role played by defects in the small intestine's tight junctions in inflammatory diseases such as those of the intestine, type 1 diabetes, allergies and asthma. Studies have also shown intestinal hyper-permeability in cases of atopic eczema[20] and asthma.[21]

Dr. Seignalet tested his hypotoxic diet on eighty-five patients who had been suffering from asthma for varying periods. In eighty patients, the disease went into complete or quasi-complete remission after a few weeks or a few months. These patients no longer take any medication at all or, in very rare cases, take only small doses as needed. However, one of these patients, whose illness had been in remission for four years, suffered asthma again. Three patients saw improvements: crises were less frequent and less intense, respiratory abilities increased between crises and doses of medication were reduced. In two cases, the diet was a failure.

12

DRUGS USED TO TREAT
INFLAMMATORY DISEASE

1. ANTI-INFLAMMATORY
DRUGS: GENERALITIES AND
MODES OF ACTION

There are currently no drugs capable of stopping the progression of
or healing chronic inflammatory diseases. Consequently, the primary objective of medication is to treat the pain caused by this type
of disease, given the considerable effects on affected individuals'
quality of life. But the cause of these diseases is not known, and the
problem with anti-inflammatory drugs stems from that fact.

The pharmaceutical industry concentrates on symptoms and on
the development of painkillers. Generally, these drugs attempt to
reduce the collateral damage resulting from an excess of arachidonic acid, an essential fatty acid present in cellular membranes
and produced by our bodies. Arachidonic acid is a precursor of
eicosanoids, the first hormones secreted by living beings. Each cell
in an organism can produce eicosanoids. These primitive hormones

regulate our whole body, particularly our immune and reproductive systems, brain, heart and entire gastrointestinal system.[1] Eicosanoids participate in the different processes that lead to the classic signs of inflammation.

Normally, inflammation is a beneficial process for the body, as it triggers the immune system to fight against infections, repair tissues and reestablish the functioning of the infected or damaged site.[2] The inflammatory process usually regulates itself with the help of feedback mechanisms like the secretion of anti-inflammatory messenger molecules. Thus, well-controlled inflammatory responses are essential for the maintenance of good health and for homeostasis. Pathologic inflammation implies a loss of immune tolerance or of the regulatory process, which allows disease to become established, and inflammation to become chronic.

Hyperalgesia (that is, the very intense pain that often accompanies chronic inflammatory diseases) is provoked by an eicosanoid called prostaglandin E_2. This prostaglandin increases the sensitivity of receptors located on peripheral sensory neurons resident at the site of inflammation. Peripheral sensory neurons are those which, for example, are situated in the synovial fluid of the affected joint; sensory neurons of the central nervous system play an equally active role.[3] Prostaglandin E_2 acts in a very complex manner, for it acts as a pro-inflammatory mediator and also induces anti-inflammatory responses.[4] These diverse activities of prostaglandin E_2 are governed by four receptors that act differently in the transmission of signals, depending on their localization in the different tissues and the regulation of their expression. Some of these receptors will increase inflammation, as may be the case in joints, while others will protect the intestines against inflammation. Given the complexity of the action of prostaglandin E_2, it's easy to understand that anti-inflammatory drugs that target the functioning of these molecules can have unintended secondary effects, as has been the case with Vioxx and similar drugs.

2. THE MAJOR CLASSES OF PAINKILLERS
Corticosteroids

Corticosteroids are the most potent painkillers. They are artificially synthesized molecules similar in chemical structure to hormones secreted by the adrenal glands. They prevent the release of arachidonic acid from membranes. Unfortunately, corticosteroids destroy all eicosanoids indiscriminately, whether they play a positive or negative role in inflammation. Corticosteroids, therefore, cannot be administered for long periods because they can provoke serious side effects, among which are the weakening of the immune system, cognitive issues, insulin resistance, myopathy (a disorder of the muscular system) and osteoporosis.[5]

Opioids and cannabinoids

Opioids are a class of drugs that can be particularly efficient in relieving severe chronic pain. However, this class of drugs is very controlled because it is classed with illicit substances. Opioids are most often used only when other classes of painkillers have proven to be ineffective. They are sometimes administered in association with other classes of painkillers. The analgesic effect of opioids is based on their capacity to interact with one or several receptors that are specific to them and situated principally in the nervous system and the gastrointestinal tract. There are several classes of receptors that are specific to opioids: the principal ones are called mu, kappa and delta. Opioids have different capacities to reduce the perception of pain, depending on how they bind—with greater or lesser affinity—to one or several receptors specific to them. Opioids most often used in chronic, moderate and severe pain are buprenorphine, fentanyl, methadone, hydromorphone, morphine and oxycodone.[6]

The use of opioids for the treatment of chronic pain due to diseases other than cancer—such as osteoarthritis, rheumatoid arthritis and neuropathic pain—raises clinicians' concerns. They fear that their patients could develop physical dependence on, addiction to and tolerance towards these medications and that patients may use these drugs inappropriately. Moreover, the tight control exercised by police authorities over these drugs is a cause for concern and a complication for clinicians. Apart from the aforementioned problems, in a great percentage of patients, opioids often have secondary effects. Elderly patients, who are the major users of painkillers, are often weakened by other concomitant diseases. Thus, pharmacokinetic and pharmacodynamic analyses should be used to investigate possible kidney or liver failure in patients using opioids.

All these restrictions have resulted in an underutilization of this type of analgesic, as well as the prescription of suboptimal doses.[7] This situation is regrettable as the analgesic properties of opioids are definitely advantageous for certain patients whose pain is not controlled by other classes of analgesics. Patients are reassured by the better control of pain, the better quality of sleep and the possibility of longer-term analgesic activity achieved with opioids.[8]

The discovery of receptors specific to cannabinoids in the early 1990s made it possible to characterize them and to study some of their physiological properties. CB_1 receptors are present in certain areas of the nervous system and play a role in the modulation of pain by mechanisms different from those of other painkillers. CB_2 receptors may play a role in the inhibition of pro-inflammatory molecules.[9] As these substances have different modes of action from other painkillers, they symbolize hope for patients whose pain is not controlled by other painkillers.

Nonsteroidal anti-inflammatory drugs (NSAIDs)

All nonsteroidal anti-inflammatory drugs, including aspirin, inhibit the enzyme cyclooxygenase (COX). The COX enzyme plays a critical role in the synthesis of prostaglandins. In the early 1990s, it was shown that there are two forms of COX: COX-1 and COX-2. Traditional NSAIDs inhibit the two isoforms of COX. By inhibiting the action of prostaglandins, classic NSAIDs, which are nonselective, may erode the stomach lining, causing gastropathies in some users. However, studies have concluded that COX-2 acts only on inflammatory processes, and therefore does not affect the stomach.[10]

In order to diminish the gastrointestinal toxicity of NSAIDs, drugs called coxibs, such as Celebrex, Bextra, Prexige and Vioxx, which are considered selective inhibitors of COX-2, have been developed. Each was approved by the FDA. Their use on a larger scale showed that an abnormally high number of patients treated with Vioxx died of cardiovascular disease. Vioxx was withdrawn from the Canadian market in September 2004. In April 2005 and in October 2007 respectively, two other selective inhibitors of cyclooxygenase, Bextra and Prexige, met with the same fate. Systematic reviews and meta-analyses established that coxibs, including Celebrex, were associated with an increased risk of myocardial infarction when compared to placebos or to nonselective NSAIDs.[11] Meanwhile, in February 2005, despite the evidence of the risk of cardiovascular incidents associated with Celebrex, the FDA approved its use in the United States.[12] However, FDA evaluators have concluded on several occasions that Celebrex did not provide any gains when its risks and benefits were compared to those of other NSAIDs currently in use.[13] In fact, it has not been shown that coxibs' side effects are less harmful than those of NSAIDs.

Manufacturers use contradictory research results on the risk of cardiovascular diseases and cerebrovascular and gastrointestinal problems, and highlight those inconsistent results and the lack of knowledge of the long-term risk factors to continue to promote the use of Celebrex.[14]

In the meantime, Celebrex continues to be marketed, for there is a huge financial stake in it: the average cost of Celebrex is about thirteen times the cost of other nonselective NSAIDs.[15]

3. SIDE EFFECTS OF NSAIDs

NSAIDs are among the most-prescribed drugs in the world because of their analgesic, antipyretic (anti-fever) and anti-inflammatory properties.[16] NSAID prescriptions in the United States in 2004 were evaluated at more than $110 million.[17] NSAIDs are powerful pharmacological tools that, despite their relative safety, can have serious side effects on the digestive tract, liver, kidneys, blood, brain and lungs. Special attention must be paid to children, pregnant women and the elderly who take these drugs. In this regard, in 2009, the American Geriatrics Society revised its guidelines for the treatment of chronic pain in people aged sixty-five and above. Contrary to its earlier recommendations, the American Geriatric Society recommends a reduction in the use of NSAIDs due to several well-documented cases that provide evidence of potential side effects of these medications; these include renal failure, cerebral hemorrhage, hypertension, cardiac arrest and gastrointestinal complications.[18]

Yet, the vast majority of NSAID prescriptions are meant for people over sixty-five.[19] Unlike in younger populations, chronic pain in the elderly is often associated with other comorbidities, which, in addition to age, render the elderly more vulnerable to the secondary effects of drugs, as comorbidities can increase both a drug's pharmacokinetics (duration of the presence of a drug in the body) and its pharmacodynamics (action exercised by the drug on the body).[20] Given these facts, the American Geriatric Society concluded that before prescribing NSAIDs to patients who are more than sixty-five years old, doctors must do preliminary tests to ensure that the individual does not have any morbidity factors that would make the use of these drugs risky. In addition, tests to evaluate blood composition and the level of creatinine must be repeated within three months of starting long-term NSAID therapy.[21]

It is estimated that in the United States, NSAID-associated gastrointestinal toxicity is responsible for more than 100,000 hospitalizations and more than 16,000 deaths[22] every year. A systematic review of studies published between 1997 and 2008 shows that mortality in patients suffering from gastrointestinal bleeding or perforation was 7.4 percent in those who did not use NSAIDs, while this rate reached 20 percent in those who did.[23] Gastrointestinal problems such as damage to the mucosa, abdominal pain, nausea, heartburn and dyspepsia are present in 24 percent to 40 percent of those who use NSAIDs.[24] Risk factors for gastrointestinal bleeding associated with NSAID use include drug characteristics, dosage, duration of treatment, being elderly and history of stomach ulcers.[25] Because it is currently used for the prevention of cardiovascular and cerebrovascular diseases, the use of aspirin in association with other NSAIDs is a risk factor for gastrointestinal bleeding because of its anticoagulant action, which is counter to the action of blood platelets, which are responsible for blood clotting.[26]

All NSAIDs except aspirin can favor the development of cardiovascular disease.[27] Selective NSAIDs (meaning selective inhibitors of COX-2) increase the risk of blood-clot formation. The risk of cardiovascular disease is equally associated with the use of nonselective NSAIDs, particularly in patients who already take aspirin to prevent coronary and cerebrovascular disease; interferences are possible, given aspirin's antiplatelet effect. Research suggests that COX-2 inhibitors may have a cardiovascular toxicity, which may give rise to thromboses. Meta-analyses affirm the cardiotoxicity of selective inhibitors of COX-2 and nonselective NSAIDs, even though it has not yet been demonstrated. However, the risks of coronary problems caused by nonselective NSAIDs are relatively low, particularly when compared to other risk factors.[28]

Studies show that the toxic effects of NSAIDs on the liver are rarely observed in the general population.[29] However, NSAIDs carry risks for people who have liver problems such as hepatitis C, liver diseases, cirrhosis or kidney failure.[30] Whether selective or nonselective, NSAIDs have been associated with kidney-toxicity issues.

These issues can include kidney failure, which can advance to necrosis and to a possibly fatal nephrotic syndrome. Administration of NSAIDS is not recommended for individuals who suffer from kidney failure (even mildly), or from hypertension and cardiac congestion. If the side effects of nonselective NSAIDS have been well characterized, those associated with selective inhibitors of COX-2 are less well documented. However, Vioxx seemingly had deleterious effects on the kidneys, while Celebrex would less likely have such effects.[31]

Side effects from NSAIDS on the central nervous system are rare in the general population, but more common in the elderly. Tinnitus can be a sign of a high concentration of drugs in the blood. Psychoses and cognitive changes following the use of anti-inflammatory drugs are more common in the elderly and are often associated with the use of Indomethacin (Indocid). Other rare but potential side effects of NSAIDS include confusion, depression and dizziness.[32]

Aspirin and other NSAIDS can provoke respiratory problems. The most common side effect is respiratory-disease exacerbation due to the triggering of symptoms of broncho-constriction and rhinitis. This is not an allergic phenomenon. It occurs at a rate of about 0.07 percent in the general population and reaches 21 percent in adults with asthma.[33]

Ultimately, the consumption of anti-inflammatory drugs is not a harmless act, and their administration should be personalized depending on risk factors such as age and the presence of weakness or of disease that affects the different organ systems. According to Dr. T. Colin Campbell, professor emeritus in the Department of Nutritional Biochemistry at Cornell University, new drugs present even higher potential hazards since 20 percent of them have serious and unpredictable side effects. Consequently, more than 100,000 Americans die each year because they take drugs that have been prescribed to them, despite following the instructions correctly.[34]

13

ATTEMPTS TO EXPLAIN THE LACK OF CONSENSUS ON USING TARGETED NUTRITION TO PREVENT AND TREAT MANY CHRONIC DISEASES (DESPITE THE PUBLICATION OF NUMEROUS CONVINCING STUDIES)

The health systems of Western countries are very efficient in the treatment of acute diseases and emergencies such as heart attacks, cancers, fractures, trauma and infections. However, this kind of health system, based primarily on drugs and surgery, is less or not at all efficient for the treating of chronic disease. It neglects the importance of prevention—and, hence, nutrition and lifestyle—in the maintenance of good health. Because of this, the "medical world" has ignored how important nutrition could be as medication. (Yet Hippocrates, the father of medicine, born in 490 BC, affirmed, "Let food be your only drug.") It is not easy for the vast majority of individuals, including health professionals, to make pertinent and informed decisions regarding the choice of a diet likely to prevent and to treat chronic diseases.

Part of the problem stems from how little our physicians are trained in nutrition. A summary of a report that the Royal College of Physicians published in 2002[1] criticized the lack of nutrition training for medical students. The report ruled that despite the fact that the importance of diet in the maintenance of good health has been recognized in clinical medicine for several decades, most medical programs offer minimal training on nutrition. The report also mentioned the lack of coordination between different disciplines and nutrition, which was not recognized as a clinical entity related to health problems. In addition, it pointed out that the role of model diets in the prevention and treatment of diseases was greatly underestimated and that, in general, this field of expertise was not considered "true medicine." This was because clinical professors have little or no knowledge of nutrition and tend not to teach it. The report concluded that for these reasons, numerous physicians neglect clinical nutrition because they lack knowledge of the potential benefits linked to this science.

Dr. Campbell[2] reported one very surprising fact: The Danone Institute, the National Cattlemen's Beef Association, the National Dairy Council, Nestle Nutrition Institute, the Wyeth-Ayerst laboratories, the Bristol-Myers Squibb company, Baxter Healthcare and others worked together to develop a nutrition program for American medical schools. That companies and lobbyists with financial interests in the nutrition and health sectors may develop such a program and, furthermore, that in 2003, 112 American medical faculties were using this program, is questionable, to say the least.

1. OTHER OPPOSITION TO NUTRITIONAL CHANGE

If it is true that the hypotoxic diet requires real sacrifices, particularly in the beginning—changing one's eating habits is hardly ever easy—probably the most serious obstacle is that generally speaking, milk products and cereals are central pieces of our diet. Do not underestimate the emotional ties that bind individuals to the foods they've been used to eating from childhood: the current trend of "comfort foods" is indicative of this phenomenon. Possibly the major obstacle to a change in diet is the fact that the health benefits of milk products and cereals are so praised in advertising that it is difficult to go against this flow. Speaking on this subject, one American, Dr. Caldwell B. Esselstyn Jr., a very great cardiac surgeon who became the champion for treating heart and other diseases through diet, said, "Wherever you go, 99 percent of people do not eat well. The numbers are against you. It is really difficult for all these people to look at the one who is part of the 1 percent and to acknowledge that that one is right and that they are wrong."[3]

Another major obstacle is that as a whole, medical authorities believe that it is necessary to consume milk products and cereals daily. Currently, even if several studies have demonstrated the harmfulness of animal-milk consumption and the multiple health problems linked to cereal consumption in a significant percentage of individuals, the "medical establishment" and our governments do not seem concerned about the problem. In addition, though more and more people have begun to incriminate trans fats, saturated fats, refined sugar and salt as causes of obesity and chronic diseases, many governments have not yet passed laws that require food manufacturers to modify their recipes.

2. WHY IS IT DIFFICULT AND EVEN THREATENING FOR HEALTHCARE PROFESSIONALS TO BE USING DIET AS A TREATMENT FOR CHRONIC DISEASES?

According to Dr. T. Colin Campbell, "almost everything is governed by the golden rule, that is, he who has the gold establishes the rules."[4] The financial health of wealthy food and drug companies depends on them exercising control over the information that the public receives about food and health. Dr. Campbell, who has worked within the American health system at the very top levels, affirms that "science is not always the honest search for truth that so many believe it to be. It far too often involves money, power, ego and protection of personal interests above the common good. [. . .] It's not a Hollywood story; it's just day-to-day government, science and industry in the United States."[5]

Health and food companies are among the most influential organizations in the world. Kraft has annual revenue of about $30 billion. The Danone Group, an international milk-product company, has annual revenue of $15 billion. McDonald's has annual revenue of more than $15 billion.[6] According to figures from 1999, total expenses on food—including food bought by individuals, the government and businesses—exceed $700 billion annually. The pharmaceutical company Pfizer recorded $32 billion in revenue in 2002. The same year, Eli Lilly had revenue of $11 billion, while Johnson & Johnson achieved sales totaling $36 billion. In addition, several associations with hundreds of millions of dollars, such as the United Dairy Industry Association, as well as meat, egg and cereal producers, strive to promote the sales of their products and to increase their share of the market.

One way to accomplish their goals is to promote the benefits of the food products and medications that they sell. The science of food and medication then becomes a "marketing" issue. These associations form committees made up of physicians, scientific researchers and other specialists to keep an eye on American research programs that are likely to cause them trouble or be an obstacle. These scientists act as medical specialists in the media and provide data to support the health benefits of medication and foods like milk and cereals.[7]

It sometimes happens that the integrity of scientists is strongly tested by pharmaceutical companies and even universities, who usually depend on industry subsidies. For example, one university researcher saw his career compromised when, during a study, he discovered that a certain drug could cause serious side effects and was ineffective. A scientist who had highlighted the possible side effects of antidepressants lost an opportunity for employment at the University of Toronto.[8] Dr. Marcia Angell, former editor-in-chief of the *New England Journal of Medicine,* wrote a very critical article entitled "Is Academic Medicine for Sale?"[9] She stated that the tens of billions of dollars that drug companies provide physicians with each year most likely "affect the results of research, the way medicine is practiced, and even the definition of what constitutes a disease. Researchers serve as consultants to companies whose products they are studying, join advisory boards and speakers' bureaus, enter into patent and royalty arrangements, agree to be the listed authors of articles ghostwritten by interested companies, promote drugs and devices at company-sponsored symposiums, and allow themselves to be plied with expensive gifts and trips to luxurious settings. Many also have equity interests in the companies."[10]

3. METHODS OF SUBSIDY DISTRIBUTION FOR GOVERNMENT RESEARCH

The U.S. government through the National Institutes of Health subsidizes 80 percent to 90 percent of all biomedical and nutritional research studies done in U.S. universities. Despite the proven link between nutrition and health, only 3.6 percent of a budget of $24 billion from the National Institutes of Health has been assigned to studies related to nutrition and 2.4 percent to prevention programs.[11] In reality, funds allocated to prevention and nutrition are used for drugs and food supplements. In short, the majority of biomedical research studies subsidized by Americans are geared towards discovering products that the pharmaceutical industry can produce and market.[12] According to Campbell, "this litany of research on drugs, genes, devices and technology research *will never cure our chronic diseases.* Our chronic diseases are largely the result of infinitely complex assaults on our bodies resulting from the consumption of bad food. No single chemical intervention will ever equal the power of consuming the healthiest food. In addition, isolated chemicals in drug form can be very dangerous." To conclude, Campbell asks the following question: "So why is our government ignoring the abundant scientific research supporting a dietary approach in favor of largely ineffective, potentially dangerous drug and device interventions?"

4. PHARMACEUTICAL COMPANIES' GRIP ON HEALTHCARE

Many facts reported by Dr. Campbell eloquently show the major grip pharmaceutical companies and the food industry have on American healthcare. Since the same companies, most often multinationals, control healthcare in North America, and sometimes in the whole world, we are all under the same constraints. Two articles written in the journal *Protégez-vous* in May 2010[13] by Rémi Maillard confirm the important influence these companies have on our healthcare systems. The first article, about the drug and pharmaceutical industries, is titled "Marketing sur ordonnance" (which translates literally to "marketing of prescriptions"), and the second, about drug clinical trials, is titled "La grande manipulation" (which translates literally to "the great manipulation"). The first article reports that normal life events are being medicalized and benign ailments are being transformed into diseases. According to Dr. Marc Zaffran, visiting researcher at the Research Ethics Board at the University of Montreal at the time, this strategy "guarantees a large, easily extendable market" for the products of pharmaceutical companies. He suggests that the goal of pharmaceutical companies is to convert each one of us into a long-term pill consumer. He also reports some abnormalities that bring into question the independence of some specialized doctors with respect to pharmaceutical companies: for example, the fact that 95 of the 170 experts of the American Psychiatric Association who were involved in the last publication of the *Diagnostic and Statistical Manual of Mental Disorders (DSM)*—the psychiatrist's bible in North America and Europe—had financial ties to the pharmaceutical industry could be at the very least questionable. Also, pharmaceutical companies' practice of extending a patent's lifetime by slightly modifying an old drug in order to sell it at a higher price could be ethically questionable. According to Marc-André Gagnon, a researcher at the Centre for Intellectual Property Policy at McGill University (Montreal), citing a study by the independent review *Prescribe,* states that "of the 109 new molecules put on the French market in 2009, 3 represented a minor therapeutic advancement, 95 brought nothing new, 19 were squarely judged dangerous for public health and 11 were not evaluated" as reported in "Marketing sur ordonnance." In fact, according to experts consulted, drug-evaluation criteria should be better controlled so that only drugs with real therapeutic effects are subsidized by public healthcare insurance.

5. MARKETING AND R&D:
IMPACT ON MEDICINE

The article "Marketing sur ordonnance" also reports that in 2004, American pharmaceutical companies spent $61 billion on advertising—double their R&D expenditure (it seems these proportions are the same in Canada).[14] This suggests that it is not only the cost of research that determines the high price of some drugs. Moreover, in the same article, according to Dr. Alain Vadeboncoeur, head of Emergency Care Service at Montreal Heart Institute and vice president of Quebec Doctors for Medicare in 2010, the intense marketing of drugs could run "from the commercial financing of universities to biased clinical trials, from pseudo scientific publications to regular reduction of the thresholds of some disease risk factors, from the continuing education of doctors to the unceasing visits of pharmaceutical representatives with free samples. This also includes conference financing, paid meals and conference dinners in major restaurants." Still, according to him, the problem could lie in part with the state's growing lack of interest in the world of medicine, "which gives private companies a free for all pass in areas as strategic as scientific research and medical doctor continuing education." All this, as reported in the same article, could have a non-negligible effect on medical doctors because, according to Dr. Pierre Biron, a Quebec expert in drug-safety monitoring, "this influence limits their autonomy, reduces the usefulness of their prescriptions and weakens public health by increasing drug consumption."

6. NON-RECOMMENDED USE OF DRUGS AND INSUFFICIENT STUDY OF DRUG SIDE EFFECTS

An important point examined in "Marketing sur ordonnance" (*Protégez-vous*[15]) is the use of some drugs for purposes other than those specified for the drug. This practice applies to 20 percent to 50 percent of prescription drugs in the United States and Canada. In the U.S. in 2004, Pfizer spent $450 million to settle lawsuits because Neurotin, a drug meant to treat seizures, was advertised to medical doctors for non-authorized uses such as the treatment of bipolar disorder and headaches. Marketing this drug brought the company $2.8 billion in 2003. In fact, between 2004 and 2009, unethical practices by pharmaceutical companies were so frequent that seven of them paid more than $7 billion in settlements and fines.

As reported in the second article, "La grande manipulation," it appears that the pharmaceutical industry does not make enough effort to check the side effects of drugs and sometimes even hides existing data. Unfavorable clinical trials on Vioxx, the anti-inflammatory drug commercialized by Merck, were hidden, and the company was accused of causing 138,000 heart attacks in the U.S.,[16] of which 55,000 were fatal.

Fortunately, as indicated in "Marketing sur ordonnance," pockets of resistance could be organizing to counteract the increasing influence of "big pharma" on healthcare. Medical associations are requesting that gifts from the industry to physicians be refused. The American Medical Students Association led a campaign entitled PharmFree, seeking stricter regulation of the pharmaceutical business in medical schools and campuses. They are requesting that researchers publicly disclose their financial ties with companies. For several years now, most scientific journals have required researchers to reveal, at the end of their articles, all relationships that could compromise their independence. Medical students and health professionals from the University of Montreal founded the Comité de lutte anti-marketing pharmaceutique (anti-pharmaceutical marketing committee). This group requests the adoption of stricter measures against the influence of firms in universities and university health centers.[17]

EPILOGUE

We know that chronic inflammatory diseases develop in individuals with a genetic predisposition to them. However, genetic vulnerabilities manifest themselves only if one or more environmental factors encourage the expression of these genes. Even if we cannot modify our genes, at least we can act on the environmental factors—such as nutrition—that play a central role in the development of numerous chronic inflammatory diseases. It should go without saying that to maintain good health, we must both follow a diet that is properly adapted to our genes and engage in regular physical activity.

According to the American professor T. Colin Campbell, a scientist who has been at the forefront of nutrition research for more than forty years now, there are a great number of extremely serious studies supporting the hypothesis that an optimal diet can not only prevent but also treat a great variety of chronic diseases, such as cardiovascular diseases, type 2 diabetes and autoimmune diseases. According to Dr. Campbell, an optimal diet should be based on whole, unrefined foods, including legumes, whole grains, fresh fruits and vegetables, as well as on an avoidance of milk products, a reduced consumption of meat, sugar, salt and fats, and as far as possible, a reduced consumption of industrially produced foods.[1]

The diet recommended by Dr. Seignalet is generally the same as the one Dr. Campbell recommends, with very few exceptions. Dr. Seignalet recommends the elimination of almost all cereals in individuals suffering from chronic inflammatory diseases; his hypotoxic (or ancestral) diet distinguishes itself from others by its basis on the hypothesis that the dietary lifestyle that preceded the development of agriculture about 10,000 years ago was better adapted to human digestive enzymes than the dietary lifestyle that followed it. For millions of years, our ancestors, and later *Homo sapiens,* exclusively consumed wild animals and non-cultivated plants, which fashioned the physiology of their digestive systems, including their digestive enzymes. According to Seignalet, the change in eating habits to a predominance of cereals and milk products could have caused a conflict between our old genes and the new diet. This is very plausible, given that 10,000 years represent less than 1 percent of humankind's history of evolution. This conflict may also be responsible for metabolic acidosis (acidification of body fluids), which is a cause of numerous chronic inflammatory diseases in the West. Metabolic acidosis is a consequence of the reduced amount of potassium in the modern diet, a reduction that is promoted by consumption of very large quantities of cereals, milk products and meats and a low consumption of plants. The latter are the major sources of potassium.

Seignalet's theory takes another important point equally into consideration—cooking certain foods, particularly animal protein and cereals containing gluten at high temperatures (= 120°C or 248°F) causes Maillard-molecule formation. Maillard molecules, made up of different glycotoxins, are formed following nonenzymatic reactions between amino acids and sugars or lipids when they are subjected to high temperatures. In fact, Seignalet's decision to eliminate cereals seemed more like the fruit of intuition and observation rather than of exact knowledge of the processes responsible for these biochemical reactions. It is really only since

2003, the year Seignalet passed away, that two important discoveries have made it possible to stress the particularly negative effects of glycotoxins—formed by cooking foods at high temperature—in the development of chronic diseases. The first discovery made it possible to highlight the presence of acrylamide in commonly consumed foods, like the majority of cereals used in making bread, pasta and other flour-based foods, and potatoes when they are cooked at high temperatures, as is the case with fries and chips. Acrylamide is a glycotoxin variant that is particularly dangerous for certain tissues that renew themselves slowly. The formation of acrylamide in cereals and potatoes is due to the presence of large quantities of free asparagine, an amino acid that transforms into acrylamide in the presence of sugar or starch when foods are cooked at a high temperature—as is the case with fries, chips and cooked cereal products. The second discovery concerns the identification of RAGEs on the surface of some of our cells. RAGEs recognize glycotoxins and bind to them in a specific manner, which induces inflammation, compromises the normal functioning of cells and causes the development of chronic disease.

It is clear that Seignalet's choice to eliminate a majority of cereals from his hypotoxic diet is now justified by solid scientific arguments based on controlled experiments (see chapters 3 and 4) as well as on extremely positive results that this physician researcher obtained by putting patients on his diet. For example, the greater majority of rheumatoid arthritis patients who correctly followed the hypotoxic diet saw their pain completely disappear and their disease put into remission, as did the sufferers of ninety other chronic diseases. We clearly do not refer here to a cure but to remission, since the disease returns if the patient stops following the diet. Despite Dr. Seignalet's death in 2003, several people have continued to testify on the Internet that their chronic disease completely disappeared and that they recovered their health by following the hypotoxic diet. In addition, since the publication of the French version of my book in May 2011, I have received on my blog (jacquelinelagace.net) hundreds of testimonials demonstrating the effectiveness of the hypotoxic diet in inducing remission of the majority of chronic inflammatory diseases.

Given the extraordinary and unexpected results that I personally obtained by following the hypotoxic diet, I must say that it was with ever-increasing interest that I spent more than two years of my life writing this book and conducting an exhaustive review of the scientific literature with the goal of verifying the solidity of the scientific basis of Dr. Seignalet's hypotoxic diet. I take this opportunity to pay homage to Dr. Seignalet who, despite his very limited financial resources and the sometimes wild opposition to his work, showed creativity, boldness and exceptional courage in his quest for a diet that could help an increasing number of chronic inflammatory disease sufferers.

It is encouraging to see that currently in the medical world, there is an emerging awareness, albeit a timid one, of the phenomenon of pain. I present as proof an article from the newspaper *La Presse* from July 2010.[2] There is a report in this newspaper that states that at Hôtel-Dieu (which is part of the Hospital of the University of Montreal), a course is now offered for individuals suffering from chronic pain; and, for the first time, Montreal was the host (in August 2010) of the 13th World Congress on Pain. In recent decades, chronic pain has become a more and more rampant phenomenon, currently affecting more than 20 percent of Canadians.[3] We hope that the emerging awareness of chronic pain will make it possible for Dr. Seignalet's teachings to reach many more people, help them recover their health and rid them of unbearable pain.

Generally, Dr. Seignalet's ancestral diet is first of all meant for individuals already suffering from chronic inflammatory diseases. However, a diet that contains very few toxic glycotoxins would be beneficial for all as a preventive measure, and more particularly for the majority of individuals above age fifty. Our excretory organs and our eliminatory systems get less efficient with age, and the majority of people risk developing at least one of the diseases promoted by bad nutrition: arthritis, heart diseases, type 2 diabetes and cancer. The social and economic costs borne by our society of treating often avoidable chronic diseases are enormous. These costs, which are already very heavy and ever-increasing, should push our governments to require the food industry to modify its recipes, taking into account recent knowledge about proper nutrition to preserve the capital health of the population. For example, among other possibilities, the neutralization or the elimination of asparagine, the amino acid that in association with sugars is responsible for the formation of acrylamide in bread, pasta, chips, fried potatoes and many foods cooked at high temperatures, should not be a challenge that the food industry cannot overcome (see chapter 4 section 7).

There is hope, for the public is now better informed and has access to information sources such as the Internet. Maybe even more important is that people are increasingly aware that our health system generates outrageous costs and that these costs keep increasing every year. Parallel to rising costs, it is also evident that our health system suffers an almost unmanageable congestion, partly due to the rising tide of chronic disease. As we have reached a point where consumption of harmful food products and our sedentary lifestyle seriously endanger the survival of our healthcare system, a significant part of the population seems to be aware of this enormous problem and is willing to admit that not only can a targeted diet prevent diseases, it can also treat a great number of chronic diseases.

Changing our nutritional habits is no longer a matter of choice but one of necessity. Where toxic substances in mass-produced foods are concerned, it is the population who must demand that our governments take responsibility and require the food and pharmaceutical industries to stop solely targeting profits and start catering to the health of the people by adopting ethical and responsible behavior.

GLOSSARY

ACETAMINOPHEN (E.G., TYLENOL): Analgesic and antipyretic drug; therefore acts against pain and fever. It has no anti-inflammatory activity.

ALLELE: One of the various forms that the same gene can take.

ALLOANTIGENS: *Allo*—Greek word meaning "other" or "different." Immunologically speaking, individuals from the same species are different, except for true twins or homozygotes.

ANGIOGENESIS: The physiological process involving the growth of new blood vessels from pre-existing vessels. Angiogenesis is a normal and vital process in growth and development, as well as in wound healing and in granulation tissue. However, it is also a fundamental step in the transition of tumors from dormancy to malignancy.

ANTIBODY: Immunoglobulin protein that recognizes a particular antigenic site called epitope. Antibodies facilitate the elimination of antigens. Membrane antibodies are expressed at the surface of B lymphocytes that have not encountered antigens specific to them (naive B lymphocytes).

ANTIGENS: Comes from the word *anti,* which means "against," and from the word *generate.* In immunology, the term antigen designates any molecule able to trigger an immune response capable of neutralizing or destroying the antigenic molecule.

APOPTOSIS: Programmed cell death; that is, cell suicide triggered by a signal. This activity is particularly beneficial for abnormal or cancer cells.

AUTO-ANTIBODIES: Antibodies fighting against self-antigens or the individual's own tissues.

AXON: Long cylindrical projection of a neuron that enables the flow of nervous impulses.

CALCIDIOL: Intermediary molecule of vitamin D.

CALCITRIOL: Hormone synthesized from vitamin D by the kidneys and liver. It increases the level of calcium in the blood and promotes bone formation.

CANNABINOIDS: Molecules present in cannabis that act on certain cells via the intermediary of specific receptors. May play a role in pain modulation and the inhibition of pro-inflammatory molecules.

CASEIN: Set of principal milk proteins. These molecules are precipitated from milk at pH = 4.6, whereas proteins dubbed whey remain in solution at this pH.

CELL LYSIS: Dissolution or destruction of the structure of a cell or bacterium.

COLLAGEN: Fibrous protein, main constituent of connective tissue.

C-REACTIVE PROTEIN: Protein present in serum during the inflammatory phase. This protein can be linked to bacterial cell walls to favor their phagocytosis.

COMMENSAL BACTERIA OR FLORA: Microorganisms that live at the expense of another organism without causing it any damage. They could even be beneficial to the host organism.

CREATININE: Substance containing nitrogen that is eliminated by the kidneys. A high concentration of creatinine in the blood indicates that the kidneys are not functioning properly and are therefore incapable of efficiently eliminating waste and drugs.

CYTOKINES: Small peptides mainly secreted by immune system cells that play a role as messengers by modulating immune reactions. Cytokines act on other cells through receptors specific to them found on the target cells they modify.

DERMATITIS HERPETIFORMIS: Chronic and benign skin condition, characterized by itching and an intense burning sensation.

DIARTHRODIAL JOINT: Movable joint with a capsule (e.g., the knee).

DNA (DEOXYRIBONUCLEIC ACID): Molecule carrying hereditary genetic information in the form of genes that make up chromosomes in the cell nucleus.

EICOSANOIDS: Pro-inflammatory molecules derived from fatty acids that are very powerful chemical mediators locally involved in inflammation. Prostaglandins are eicosanoids.

ENSILAGE: Fodder preservation process that requires airtight bacterial fermentation, which leads to an acidic fodder.

ENTEROCYTE: Cylindrical cell of the intestinal epithelium with a flattened extremity covered with microvilli.

ENTEROVIRUS: Virus that enters the human body through the gastro-intestinal system and that is strictly confined to it. They are capable of living outside the body for a long time.

ENZYMES: Proteins that trigger biochemical reactions.

ESSENTIAL MICRONUTRIENTS: Some amino acids, fatty acids, vitamins and some minerals that need to be obtained from the diet because the human body cannot produce them or produces them at quantities lower than needed by normal human metabolism.

EXCRETORY ORGANS: Organs that evacuate waste or harmful substances: the liver, the kidneys, the lungs, the skin, the mucosa and the intestine.

FDA (FOOD AND DRUG ADMINISTRATION): American government agency in charge of drug monitoring.

FREE RADICALS: Unstable oxygen molecules that try to link up to an organism's molecules or cells, leading to its disruption or destruction, just as rust does to a metal. Free radicals can come to us from our lifestyle: an unbalanced diet, stress, pesticides, pollution, etc. Free radicals can be neutralized by antioxidants present in food.

GERMS: Generic, nonscientific word used to designate viruses, bacteria and all microscopic organisms.

GLYCEMIC INDEX: Measure of the blood sugar level after ingestion of carbohydrates.

GLYCOPROTEIN: Molecular compound resulting from the bonding of a protein to a carbohydrate (sugar).

HISTOCOMPATIBILITY: Ability of tissues to coexist. The degree of histocompatibility between the major antigens of two individuals makes it possible to predict if a transplant will be accepted. If the degree of compatibility is low, the transplant will be rejected.

HLA (HUMAN LEUKOCYTE ANTIGEN): Genetic term used to designate the human major histocompatibility complex responsible for the recognition of self and nonself.

IGF-1: Growth factor whose molecular structure is similar to that of insulin.

INFLAMMATION: Local accumulation of liquid, plasmatic protein and white blood cells from blood vessels.

INSULIN INDEX: Measure of the insulin level after ingestion of a food item.

INSULINEMIA: Blood insulin level.

INSULIN RESISTANCE: A state of excess insulin.

IU (INTERNATIONAL UNIT): Measurement unit of the amount of a substance based on its biological effects.

INTESTINAL HYPERPERMEABILITY: Leaking of the intestinal mucosa allowing the passage of an excess of big molecules that were insufficiently digested by enzymes.

ISOMERS: Compounds with the same molecular formula but with different spatial organization, hence the possibility of different reactions.

LIPOPOLYSACCHARIDE: Molecule found in the external membrane of the cell wall of gram-negative bacteria and made up of a lipid and a polysaccharide (sugar).

LONGITUDINAL STUDY: Study that enables the measurement of an effect in a group of patients at different moments in time.

LYMPH: White extracellular liquid from the blood that accumulates in tissues. Lymph is carried back by lymphatic vessels across the lymphatic system and all the way to the thoracic channel, where it returns into the bloodstream.

MACULAR DEGENERATION: Progressive destruction of the macula, the most light-sensitive point of the retina, which is the point corresponding to the maximal visual acuity.

META-ANALYSIS: Statistical analysis procedure whereby results from a series of independent studies on the same subject are combined to reach a general conclusion that each of these studies could not reach independently.

METABOLIC ACIDOSIS: Excess production of acidity or the kidneys' failure to eliminate this acidity.

MOLECULAR MIMICRY: Phenomenon in which a microorganism has an antigen that strongly resembles the antigen of the host. Molecular mimicry can provoke an autoimmune disease.

MONOZYGOTIC TWINS: Genetically identical twins coming from the same egg fertilized by one sperm. The egg was divided into two during the initial developmental phases, giving two distinct but genetically identical individuals.

MUCINS: Various strongly glycosylated surface proteins. They play a role as ligands; that is, they are able to link with specific receptors. These proteins are part of the viscous solutions that act as protective lubricants of internal and external body surfaces.

MYELIN: Protective lipid sheath in nervous tissues.

NARCOLEPSY: Neurologic disease with daily episodes of irresistible sleep attacks.

NEOPLASIA: Pathological proliferation of cells or tissues leading to the formation of a tumor.

NEUROTOXICITY: Impact of a poison or a harmful substance on the nervous system.

OLIGO ELEMENTS: Elements needed in very small quantities, such as some dietary minerals like selenium, for which the required quantity is 200 micrograms per day (0.002 g/day), compared to calcium, for which the daily consumption should be 1 gram. Large quantities of selenium are toxic. About ninety of the minerals derived from soil are essential.

OPIOIDS: Drugs derived from opium for pain reduction.

OXIDATIVE STRESS: Attacks on cellular constituents through oxidation reactions, just as oxygen in the air can oxidize iron.

PARATHORMONE: Hormone secreted by the parathyroid glands found above the adrenal glands. This hormone works in concert with vitamin D to increase intestinal absorption of calcium when there is an acid-base equilibrium in the body. However, when the level of acidity in body fluids is too high, this leads to an excess secretion of parathyroid hormone, which has an opposite effect, inducing demineralization and resorption of bone, hence promoting osteoporosis in the elderly.

PATHOGENESIS: Mechanism by which a disease is caused.

PERISTALSIS: Wavelike intestinal movement that reduces the diameter of the digestive tube in a sequential manner to slowly move food from one end to the other in the same direction.

PH: Hydrogen potential or pH is a measure of the concentration of hydrogen ions (H^+) in a solution. The pH of body fluids is particularly important and it is indispensable for life that blood pH be maintained at a slightly alkaline level between 7.3 and 7.4.

PHAGOCYTOSIS: Ingestion of particles or microorganisms by cells such as macrophages and neutrophilic leukocytes. There are vesicles in macrophages that contain enzymes able to digest pathogens into small molecules.

PHARMACODYNAMICS: The study of the action of drugs on healthy organisms.

PHARMACOVIGILANCE (DRUG SAFETY MONITORING): The study of the unexpected side effects of new drugs.

PLACEBO: Pharmacologically inert substance used as a control to evaluate the real effects of a drug.

PROBIOTICS: Living microorganisms that improve the health of a host when administered in adequate amounts.

RANDOM FACTORS: Unpredictable factors related to chance (e.g., stress that can have an influence on the development of a disease).

SAPROPHYTIC BACTERIA: Bacteria that feed on decaying organic material while living in symbiosis with humans; that is, they provide a service to humans without being harmful.

SEDIMENTATION RATE: Nonspecific evaluation of inflammation as a function of the speed and time needed for red blood cells to settle in a tube during centrifugation.

SELF: Comprises all the antigenic molecules that determine an individual x. These antigenic molecules come from one's own genes, whereas "nonself" involves all antigenic molecules foreign to the said individual x, such as food antigens, antigens of microbial origin or antigens from all other living organisms.

SPORADIC ATAXIA: Term designating various coordination and balance issues associated with problems with the cerebellum.

SUPERANTIGENS: Very reactive antigens that do not respect the usual specificity rules in immunology. One superantigen can activate an inordinate number of cells.

SYNOVIAL FLUID: Transparent lubricating liquid secreted by the synovial membrane that carpets the internal face of mobile joint capsules.

TERATOGENIC EFFECT: Effect leading to abnormalities in a developing embryo.

TRANS-FATTY ACIDS: All unsaturated fatty acids that contain one or more isolated double bonds in the trans position.

ENDNOTES

INTRODUCTION

1. Website of the Arthritis Society.
2. J.-P. Pelletier, J. Martel-Pelletier and S.B. Abramson, "Osteoarthritis, an inflammatory disease," *Arthritis Rheum,* vol. 44, 2001, p. 1237–47.
3. J. Seignalet, *L'Alimentation ou la troisième médecine,* 5e édition, Paris, Office d'Édition Impression Librairie, 2004, 660 p.

1   THE ONSET OF PAIN, AND MY SEARCH FOR SOLUTIONS

1. B. Caldwell, S. Aldington, M. Weatherall et al., "Risk of cardiovascular events and celecoxib: A systematic review and meta-analysis," *J R Soc Med,* vol. 99, 2006, p. 132–40; <www.passeportsante.net>.

2   PUTTING THE HYPOTOXIC DIET TO THE TEST

1. www.seignalet.com.
2. J. Seignalet, *L'Alimentation ou la troisième médecine,* 5e édition, Paris, Office d'Edition Impression Librairie, 2004, 660 p.
3. R. Béliveau and D. Gingras, *Les Aliments contre le cancer,* Québec, Éditions du Trécarré, 2005, 213 p.

3   CLINICAL TESTING AND RESULTS

1. L. Vase, J.L. Riley and D.D. Price, "A comparison of placebo effects in clinical analgesic trials versus studies of placebo analgesia," *Pain,* vol. 99, 2002, p. 443–52.
2. A. Hróbjartsson and P.C. Gøtzsche, "Is the placebo powerless?" *New Engl J Med,* vol. 344, 2001, p. 1594–99.

3. L. Vase, J.L. Riley and D.D. Price, "A comparison of placebo effects in clinical analgesic trials versus studies of placebo analgesia," *Pain,* vol. 99, 2002, p. 443–52.

4. A. Hróbjartsson and P.C. Gøtzsche, "Is the placebo powerless? Update of a systematic review with 52 new randomized trials comparing placebo with no treatment," *J Intern Med,* vol. 256, 2004, p. 91–100.

5. F. Benedetti, L. Colloca, E. Torre et al., "Placebo-responsive Parkinson patients show decreased activity in single neurons of subthalamic nucleus," *Nat Neurosci,* 2004, vol. 7, p. 587–88.

6. G. Buckland, C.A. Gonzalez, A. Agudo et al., "Adherence to the Mediterranean diet and risk of coronary heart disease in the Spanish EPIC cohort study," *Am J Epidemiol,* vol. 170, 2009, p. 1518–29.

7. C.B. Esselstyn Jr., S.G. Ellis, S.V. Medendorp et al., "Updating a 12-year experience with arrest and reversal therapy for coronary disease," *Am J Cardiol,* vol. 84, 1999, p. 339–41.

8. See also T.C. Campbell and T. M. Campbell, *Le Rapport Campbell. Révélations stupéfiantes sur les liens entre L'Alimentation et la santé à long terme,* Outremont, Éditions Ariane, 2008, 488 p.

9. C.B. Esselstyn, Jr., "Resolving the coronary artery disease epidemic through plant-based nutrition," *Prev Cardiol,* vol. 4, 2001, p. 171–77.

10. www.passeportsante.net.

4 KEY ELEMENTS OF DR. SEIGNALET'S DIET

1. D. Thomas, "The mineral depletion of foods available to us as a nation 1940–2002: A review of the 6th Edition of McCance and Widdowson," *Nutr Health,* vol. 19, nos. 1–2, 2007, p. 21–55; A.N. Mayer, "Historical changes in the mineral content of fruits and vegetables," *British Food Journal,* vol. 99, 1997, 207–11.

2. R. El Asmar, p. Panigrahi, p. Bamford et al., "Host-dependent activation of the zonulin system is involved in the impairment of the gut barrier function following bacterial colonization," *Gastroenterol,* vol. 123, 2002, p. 1607–15; J. Visser, J. Rozing, A. Sapone et al., "Tight junctions, intestinal permeability and autoimmunity: Celiac disease and type 1 diabetes paradigms," *Ann NY Acad Sci,* vol. 1165, 2009, p. 195–205.

3. O. Vaarala, M.A. Atkinson and J. Neu, "The 'perfect storm' for type 1 diabetes: The complex interplay between intestinal microbiota, gut permeability, and mucosal immunity," *Diabetes,* vol. 57, 2008, p. 2555–62.

4. J. Visser, J. Rozing, A. Sapone et al., "Tight junctions, intestinal permeability and autoimmunity: Celiac disease and type 1 diabetes paradigms," *Ann NY Acad. Sci.,* vol. 1165, 2009, p. 195–205

5. A. Fasano, "Pathological and therapeutic implications of macromolecule passage through the tight junction," in *Tight Junctions,* CRC Press Inc., Boca Raton, Florida, 2001, p. 697–722; A.M. Mowat, "Anatomical basis of tolerance and immunity to intestinal antigens," *Nat Rev Immunol,* vol. 3, 2003, p. 331–41; A. Fasano, "Intestinal zonulin: Open sesame!" *Gut,* vol. 49, 2001, p. 159–62.

6. A.M. Mowat, "Anatomical basis of tolerance and immunity to intestinal antigens," *Nat Rev Immunol,* vol. 3, 2003, p. 331–41; A. Fasano, "Intestinal zonulin: Open sesame!" *Gut,* vol. 49, 2001, p. 159–62.

7. S. Gorbach and E. Bengt, "Gustafsson memorial lecture: 'Function of the normal human microflora,'" *Scand J Infect Dis,* vol. 49, 1986, p. 17–30.

8. A. Ouwehand, E. Isolauri and S. Salminen, "The role of the intestinal microflora for the development of the immune system in early chidhood," *Eur J Nutr,* vol. 41, 2002, p. 132–37.

9. J. Turner, "Molecular basis of epithelial barrier regulation: From basic mechanisms to clinical application," *Am J Pathol,* vol. 169, 2006, p. 1901–09; G. Gasbarrini and M. Montalto, "Structure and function of tight junctions: Role in intestinal barrier," *Ital J Gastroenterol Hepatol,* vol. 31, 1999, p. 481–88.

10. G. Gasbarrini and M. Montalto, "Structure and function of tight junctions: Role in intestinal barrier," *Ital J Gastroenterol Hepatol,* vol. 31, 1999, p. 481–88; A. Nusrat, J. Turner and J. Madara, "Molecular physiology and pathophysiology of tight junctions. IV. Regulation of tight junctions by extracellular stimuli: Nutrients, cytokines and immune cells," *Am J Physiol Gastrointest Liver Physiol,* vol. 279, 2000, p. G851–57.

11. Fasano, "Zonulin and its regulation of intestinal barrier function: The biological door to inflammation, autoimmunity, and cancer," *Physiol Rev,* vol. 91, 2011, 151–75.

12. A. Fasano, "Pathological and therapeutic implications of macromolecule passage through the tight junction," in *Tight Junctions,* CRC Press Inc., Boca Raton, Florida, 2001, 697–722.

13. G.S. Cooper and B.C. Stroehla, "The epidemiology of autoimmune diseases," *Autoimmun,* vol. 2, 2003, p. 119–25.

14. A. Fasano and T. Shea-Donohue, "Mechanisms of disease: The role of intestinal barrier function in the pathogenesis of gastrointestinal autoimmune diseases," *Nat Clin Pract Gastroenterol Hepatol,* vol. 2, 2005, p. 416–21.

15. A. Timmer, "Environmental influences on inflammatory bowel disease manifestations: Lessons from epidemiology," *Dig Dis,* vol. 21, 2003, p. 91–104; M.A. Feeney, F. Murphy and A.J. Clegg, "A case-control study of childhood environmental risk factors for the development of inflammatory bowel disease," *Eur J Gastroenterol Hepatol,* vol. 14, 2002, p. 529–34.

16. H. Asakura, K. Suzuki, T. Kitahora et al., "Is there a link between food and intestinal microbes and the occurrence of Crohn's disease and ulcerative colitis?" *J Gastroenterol Hepatol,* vol. 23, 2008, p. 1794–1801.

17. Ibid.

18. Ibid.

19. T. Stefanelli, A. Malesci, A. Repici et al., "New insights into inflammatory bowel disease pathophysiology: Paving the way for novel therapeutic targets," *Curr Drug Targets,* vol. 9, 2008, p. 413–18; J. Wyatt, H. Vogelsang, W. Hubl et al., "Intestinal permeability and the prediction of relapse in Crohn's disease," *Lancet,* vol. 341, 1993, p. 1437–39.

20. J. Visser, J. Rozing, A. Sapone et al., "Tight junctions, intestinal permeability and autoimmunity: Celiac disease and type 1 diabetes paradigms," *Ann NY Acad Sci,* vol. 1165, 2009, p. 195–205; O. Vaarala, M.A. Atkinson and J. Neu, "The 'perfect storm' for type 1 diabetes: The complex interplay between intestinal microbiota, gut permeability, and mucosal immunity," *Diabetes,* vol. 57, 2008, p. 2555–62.

21. J.L. Madara and J.S. Trier, "Structural abnormalities of jejunal epithelial cell membranes in coeliac sprue," *Lab Invest,* vol. 43, 1980, p. 254–61; J.D. Schulzke, C.J. Bentzel, I. Schulzke et al., "Epithelial tight junction structure in the jejunum of children with acute and treated coeliac sprue," *Pediatr Res,* vol. 43. 1998, p. 435–41.

22. J.D. Schulzke, C.J. Bentzel, I. Schulzke et al., "Epithelial tight junction structure in the jejunum of children with acute and treated coeliac sprue," *Pediatr Res,* vol. 43. 1998, p. 435–41; A. Fasano, T. Not, W. Wang et al., "zonulin: A newly discovered modulator of intestinal permeability, and its expression in coeliac disease," *Lancet,* vol. 355, 2000, p. 1518–19.

23. M.G. Clemente, S. De Virgiliis, J.S. Kang et al., "Early effects of gliadin on enterocyte intracellular signaling involved in intestinal barrier function," *Gut,* vol. 52, 2003, p. 218–23.

24. R. D'Inca, V. Di Leo, G. Corrao et al., "Intestinal permeability test as a predictor of clinical courses in Crohn's disease," *Am J Gastroenterol,* vol. 94, 1999, p. 2956–60; E.J. Irvine and J.K. Marshall, "Increased intestinal permeability precedes the onset of Crohn's disease in a subject with familiar risk," *Gastroenterology,* vol. 119, 2000, p. 1740–44.

25. U. Christen and M.G. von Herrath, "Induction, acceleration or prevention of autoimmunity by molecular mimicry," *Mol Immunol,* vol. 40, 2004, p. 1113–20.

26. A. Fasano and T. Shea-Donohue, "Mechanisms of disease: The role of intestinal barrier function in the pathogenesis of gastrointestinal autoimmune diseases," *Nat Clin Pract Gastroenterol Hepatol,* vol. 2, 2005, p. 416–21.

27. J. Visser, J. Rozing and A. Sapone et al., "Tight junctions, intestinal permeability and autoimmunity: Celiac disease and type 1 diabetes paradigms," *Ann NY Acad Sci,* vol. 1165, 2009, p. 195–205; A. Fasano and T. Shea-Donohue, "Mechanisms of disease: The role of intestinal barrier function in the pathogenesis of gastrointestinal autoimmune diseases," *Nat Clin Pract Gastroenterol Hepatol,* vol. 2, p. 416–21.

28. O. Vaarala, M.A. Atkinson and J. Neu, "The 'perfect storm' for type 1 diabetes: The complex interplay between intestinal microbiota, gut permeability, and mucosal immunity," *Diabetes,* vol. 57, 2008, p. 2555–62.

29. L.V. Hooper, "Bacterial contributions to mammalian gut development," *Trends Microbiol,* vol. 12, 2004, p. 129–34; L.V. Hooper and J.I. Gordon, "Commensal host-bacterial relationships in the gut," *Science,* vol. 292, 2001, p. 1115–18; T.S. Stappenbeck, L.V. Hooper and J.I. Gordon, "Developmental regulation of intestinal angiogenesis by indigenous microbes via Paneth cells," *Proc Nat Acad Sci USA,* vol. 99, 2002, p. 15451–55; S.K. Mazmanian, C.H. Liu and A.O. Tzianabos et al., "An immunomodulatory molecule of symbiotic bacteria directs maturation of the host immune system," *Cell,* vol. 122, 2005, p. 107–18.

30. F.D.S. Calcinaro, M. Marinaro, P. Candeloro et al., "Oral probiotic administration induces interleukin-10 production and prevents spontaneous autoimmune diabetes in the non-obese diabetic mouse," *Diabetologia,* vol. 48, 2005, p. 1565–75.

31. J. Neu, C.M. Reverte, A.D. Mackey et al., "Changes in intestinal morphology and permeability in the biobreeding rat before the onset of type 1 diabetes," *J Pediatr Gastroenterol Nutr,* vol. 40, 2005, p. 589–95; J.B. Meddings, J. Jarand, S.J. Urbanski et al., "Increased gastrointestinal permeability is an early lesion in the spontaneously diabetic BB rat," *Am J Physiol,* vol. 276, 1999, p. G951–57.

32. M. Secondulfo, D. Iafusco, R. Carratu et al., "Ultrastructural mucosal alterations and increased intestinal permeability in non-celiac, type 1 diabetic patients," *Dig Liver Dis,* vol. 36, 2004, p. 35–45.

33. T. Watts, I. Berti, A. Sapone et al., "Role of the intestinal tight junction modulator zonulin in the pathogenesis of type 1 diabetes in BB diabetic-prone rats," *Proc Nat Acad Sci USA,* vol. 102, 2005, p. 2916–21; A. Sapone, L. de Magistris, M. Pietzak et al., "zonulin upregulation is associated with increased gut permeability in subjects with type 1 diabetes and their relatives," *Diabetes,* vol. 55, 2006, p. 1443–49.

34. E. Savilahti, T. Ormala, T. Saukkonen et al., "Jejuna of patients with insulin dependent diabetes mellitus (IDDM) show signs of immune activation," *Clin Exp Immunol,* vol. 116, 1999, p. 70–7; M. Westerholm-Ormio, O. Vaarala, p. Pihkala et al., "Immunologic activity in the small

intestinal mucosa of pediatric patients with type 1 diabetes," *Diabetes,* vol. 52, 2003, p. 2287–95; R. Auricchio, F. Paparo, M. Maglio et al., "In vitro-deranged intestinal immune response to gliadin in type 1 diabetes," *Diabetes,* vol. 53, 2004, p. 1680–83.

35. O. Vaarala, p. Klemetti, E. Savilahti et al., "Cellular immune response to cow's milk beta-actoglobulin in patients with newly diagnosed IDDM," *Diabetes,* vol. 45, 1996, p. 178–82; p. Klemetti, E. Savilahti, J. Ilonen et al., "T-cell reactivity to wheat gluten in patients with insulin-dependent diabetes mellitus," *Scand J Immunol,* vol. 47, 1998, p. 48–53.

36. R. Auricchio, F. Paparo, M. Maglio et al., "In vitro-deranged intestinal immune response to gliadin in type 1 diabetes," *Diabetes,* vol. 53, 2004, p. 1680–83.

37. M.R. Pastore, E. Bazzigaluppi, C. Belloni et al., "Six months of gluten-free diet do not influence autoantibody titers, but improve insulin secretion in subjects at high risk for type 1 diabetes," *J Clin Endocrinol Metab,* vol. 88, 2003, p. 162–65.

38. M. Oikarinen, S. Tauriainen, T. Honkanen et al., "Detection of enteroviruses in the intestine of type 1 diabetic patients," *Clin Exp Immunol,* vol. 151, 2008, p. 71–75.

39. H.K. Akerblom, S.M. Virtanen, J. Ilonen et al. (National TRIGR Study Group), "Dietary manipulation of beta cell autoimmunity in infants at increased risk of type 1 diabetes: A pilot study," *Diabetologia,* vol. 48, 2005, p. 829–37; O. Vaarala, "Leaking gut in type 1 diabetes," *Curr Op in Gastroenterol,* vol. 24, 2008, p. 701–06.

40. S. Gorbach and E. Bengt, "Gustafsson memorial lecture: Function of the normal human microflora," *Scand J Infect Dis,* vol. 49, 1986, p. 17–30.

41. M.D. Pimentel, D. Wallace, D. Hallegua et al., "A link between irritable bowel syndrome and fibromyalgia may be related to findings on lactulose breath testing," *Ann Rheum Dis,* vol. 63, 2004, p. 450–52.

42. A. Goebel, S. Buhner, R. Schedel et al., "Altered intestinal permeability in patients with primary fibromyalgia and in patients with complex regional pain syndrome," *Rheumatology,* vol. 47, 2008, p. 1223–27.

43. T.T. MacDonald and G. Monteleone, "Immunity, inflammation, and allergy in the gut," *Science,* vol. 307, 2005, p. 1920–25.

44. T.T. MacDonald and G. Monteleone, "Immunity, inflammation, and allergy in the gut," *Science,* vol. 307, 2005, p. 1920–25; W. Holden, T. Orchard and P. Worldsworth, "Enteropathic arthritis," *Rheum Dis Clin North Am,* vol. 29, 2003, p. 513–30; H. Reyes, R. Zapata, I. Hernandez et al., "Is a leaky gut involved in the pathogenesis of intrahepatic cholestasis of pregnancy?" *Hepatology,* vol. 43, 2006, p. 715–22; D.R. Clayburgh,

T.A. Barrett, Y. Tang et al., "Epithelial myosin light chain kinase-dependent barrier dysfunction mediates T cell activation-induced diarrhea in vivo," *J Clin Invest,* vol. 115, 2005, p. 2702–15.

45. W. Whitehead, O. Palsson and K. Jones, "Systematic review of the comorbidity of irritable bowel syndrome with other disorders: What are the causes and implications?" *Gastroenterology,* vol. 122, 2002, p. 1140–56.

46. M. Pimentel, E.J. Chow and H.C. Lin, "Normalization of lactulose breath testing correlates with symptom improvement in irritable bowel syndrome: A double blind, randomized, placebo-controlled study," *Am J Gastroenterol,* vol. 98, 2003, p. 412–19; M. Othman, R. Aguro and H.C. Lin, "Alterations in intestinal microbial flora and human disease," *Curr Opin Gastroenterol,* vol. 24, 2008, p. 11–16.

47. M. Othman, R. Aguro and H.C. Lin, "Alterations in intestinal microbial flora and human disease," *Curr Opin Gastroenterol,* vol. 24, 2008, p. 11–16.

48. D.J. Pattison, R.A. Harrison and D.P. Symmons, "The role of diet in susceptibility to rheumatoid arthritis: A systematic review," *J Rheumatol,* vol. 31, 2004, p. 1310–19.

49. P. Thrasyvoulos, J.M.D. Nightingale and R. Oldham, "Is rheumatoid arthritis a disease that starts in the intestine? A pilot study comparing an elemental diet with oral prednisolone," *Postgrad Med J,* vol. 83, 2007, p. 128–31.

50. L. Sköldstam, L. Larson and F.D. Lindstrom, "Effects of fasting and lactovegetarian diet on rheumatoid arthritis," *Scand J Rheumatol,* vol. 8, 1979, p. 249–55; I. Hafström, B. Ringertz, A. Spångberg et al., "A vegan diet free of gluten improves the signs and symptoms of rheumatoid arthritis: The effects on arthritis correlate with a reduction in antibodies to food antigens," *Rheumatology* (Oxford), vol. 40, 2001, p. 1175–79.

51. E. Benito-Garcia, D. Feskanich, F.B. Hu et al., "Protein, iron, and meat consumption and risk for rheumatoid arthritis: A prospective cohort study," *Arthritis Res Ther,* vol. 9, 2007, p. R16. (doi :10.1186/ar 2123).

52. P. Thrasyvoulos, J.M.D. Nightingale and R. Oldham, "Is rheumatoid arthritis a disease that starts in the intestine? A pilot study comparing an elemental diet with oral prednisolone," *Postgrad Med J,* vol. 83, 2007, p. 128–31.

53. P.C. Gøtzsche and H.K. Johansen, "Short-term low-dose corticosteroids vs. placebo and nonsteroidal anti-inflammatory drugs in rheumatoid arthritis," *Cochrane Database Syst Rev,* vol. 3, 2004, p. CD000189.

54. P. Thrasyvoulos, J.M.D. Nightingale and R. Oldham, "Is rheumatoid arthritis a disease that starts in the intestine? A pilot study comparing an elemental diet with oral prednisolone," *Postgrad Med J,* vol. 83, 2007, p. 128–31.

55. D.D. Adams, J.G. Knight, A. Ebringer, "Autoimmune diseases: Solution of the environmental, immunological and genetic components with principles for immunotherapy and transplantation," *Autoimmun Rev,* 2010 Jun, vol. 9, no. 8, p. 525-30

56. L.J. Albert, "Infection and rheumatoid arthritis: Guilt by association?" *J Rheumatol,* vol. 27, 2000, p. 564–66.

57. D.D. Adams, J.G. Knight and A. Ebringer, "Autoimmune diseases: Solution of the environmental, immunological and genetic components with principles for immunotherapy and transplantation," *Autoimmun Rev,* vol. 9, 2010, p. 525–30.

58. B.M. Holt and V. Formicola, "Hunters of the Ice Age: The biology of Upper Paleolithic people," *Am J Phys Anthropol,* vol. suppl. 47, 2008, p. 70–99; L. Cordain, S.B. Eaton, A. Sebastian et al., "Origins and evolution of the Western diet: Health implications for the 21st century," *Am J Clin Nutr,* vol. 81, 2005, p. 341–54; E. Pouydebat, P. Gorce, Y. Coppens et al., "Biomechanical study of grasping according to the volume of the object: Human versus non-human primates," *J Biomech,* vol. 42, 2009, p. 266–72.

59. L.A. Frassetto, R.C. Morris, Jr., D.E. Sellmeyer et al., "Diet, evolution and aging," *Eur J Nutr,* vol. 40, 2001, p. 200–13.

60. S.B. Eaton and S.B. Eaton III, "Paleolithic vs. modern diets: Selected pathophysiological implications," *Eur J Nutr,* vol. 39, 2000, p. 67–70.

61. L.A. Frassetto, R.C. Morris, Jr., D.E. Sellmeyer et al., "Diet, evolution and aging," *Eur J Nutr,* vol. 40, 2001, p. 200–13.

62. S.B. Eaton and S.B. Eaton III, "Paleolithic vs. modern diets: Selected pathophysiological implications," *Eur J Nutr,* vol. 39, 2000, p. 67–70.

63. Ibid.

64. L.A. Frassetto, R.C. Morris, Jr., D.E. Sellmeyer et al., "Diet, evolution and aging," *Eur J Nutr,* vol. 40, 2001, p. 200–13.

65. L. Cordain, S.B. Eaton, A. Sebastian et al., "Origins and evolution of the Western diet: Health implications for the 21st century," *Am J Clin Nutr,* vol. 81, 2005, p. 341–54.

66. B. Wood and M. Collard, "The human genus," *Science,* vol. 284, 1999, p. 65–71.

67. P.R. Shewry, "Wheat," *J Experimental Botany,* vol. 60, 2009, p. 1537–53.

68. A.S. Tatham and P.R. Shewry, "Allergy to wheat and related cereals," *Clin Exp Allergy,* vol. 38, 2008, p. 1712–26.

69. C. Feighery, "Coeliac disease," *British Med J,* vol. 29, 1999, p. 236–39.

70. L. Fry, "Dermatitis herpetiformis," in M.N. Marsh (dir.), *Coeliac disease,* Oxford, U.K, Blackwell Scientific Publications, 1992, p. 81–104.

71. A. Karell, A.S. Louka, S.J. Moodie et al., "HLA types in celiac disease patients not carrying the DQA1 heterodimer: Results from the Europeans genetics clusters on celiac disease," *Human Immununology,* vol. 64, 2003, p. 469–77.

72. P.R. Shewry, "Wheat," *J Experimental Botany,* vol. 60, 2009, p. 1537–53

73. S.L. Neuhausen, L. Steele, S. Ryan et al., "Co-occurrence of celiac disease and other autoimmune diseases in celiacs and their first degree relatives," *J Autoimmunity,* vol. 31, 2008, p. 160–65.

74. M.M. Singh and S.R. Roy, "Wheat gluten as a pathogenic factor in schizophrenia," *Science,* vol. 191, 1975, p. 401–02; A.E. Kalaydiian, W. Eaton, N. Cascella et al., "The gluten connection: The association between schizophrenia and celiac disease," *Acta Physchiatr Scandinavia,* vol. 113, 2006, p. 82–90.

75. R.P. Ford, "The gluten syndrome: A neurological disease," *Medical Hypotheses,* vol. 73, 2009, p. 438–40; E. Lionetti, R. Francavilla, P. Pavone et al., "The neurology of coeliac disease in childhood: What is the evidence? A systematic review and meta-analysis," *Dev Med Child Neurol,* vol. 52, 2010, p. 700–07.

76. M. Hadjivassiliou, R.A. Grunewald, B. Sharrack et al., "Gluten ataxia in perspective: Epidemiology, genetic susceptibility and clinical characteristics," *Brain,* vol. 126, 2003, p. 685–91; M. Hadjivassiliou, D.S. Sanders, N. Wooddroofe et al., "Gluten ataxia," *Cerebellum,* vol. 7, 2008, p. 494–98.

77. P. Humbert, F. Pelletier, B. Dreno et al., "Gluten intolerance and skin diseases," *Eur J Dermatol,* vol. 16, 2006, p. 4–11.

78. U. Wahnshaffe, J.D. Schulzke, M. Zeitz et al., "Predictors of clinical response to gluten-free diet in patients diagnosed with diarrhea-predominant irritable bowel syndrome," *Clin Gastroenterol Hepatol,* vol. 5, 2007, p. 844–50.

79. E.C. Grant, "Food allergies and migraine," *Lancet,* vol. 1, 1979, p. 66–69; J. Pascual and C. Leno, "A woman with daily headaches," *J Headache Pain,* vol. 6, 2005, p. 91–92.

80. K.J. Rix, J. Ditchfield, D.L. Freed et al., "Food antibodies in acute psychoses," *Psychological Medicine,* vol. 15, 1985, p. 347–54.

81. M. Hadjivassiliou, R.A. Grunewald and G.A.B. Davies-Jones, "Gluten sensitivity as a neurological illness," *J Neurol, Neurosurg Psychiatry,* vol. 72, 2002, p. 560–63.

82. S. Lucarelli, T. Frediani, A.M. Zingoni et al., "Food allergy and infantile autism," *Panminerva Med,* vol. 37, 1995, p. 137–41; K.L. Reichelt and A.M. Knivsberg, "The possibility and probability of a gut-to-brain connection in autism," *Ann Clin Psychiatry,* vol. 21, 2009, p. 205–11.

83. J.H. Elder, "The gluten-free, casein-free diet in autism: An overview with clinical implications," *Nut Clin Pract,* vol. 23, 2008, p. 583–88.

84. R.P. Ford, "The gluten syndrome: A neurological disease," *Medical Hypotheses,* vol. 73, 2009, p. 438–40.

85. Ibid.

86. Ibid.

87. A. Sapone, K.M. Lammers, V. Casolaro et al., "Divergence of gut permeability and mucosal immune gene expression in two gluten-associated conditions: Celiac disease and gluten sensitivity," BMC *Medicine,* vol. 9, no. 23, 2011. doi: 10.1186/1741-7015-9-23; A. Sapone, J. Bai, C. Ciacci, et al., "Spectrum of gluten-related disorders: Consensus on new nomenclature and classification," BMC *Medicine,* vol. 10, no. 13, 2012. doi: 10.1186/1741-7015-10-13.

88. H.L. McClellan, S.J. Miller and P.E. Hartmann, "Evolution of lactation: Nutrition versus protection with special reference to five mammalian species," *Nut Res Rev,* vol. 21, 2008, p. 97–116.

89. S. Kamiński, A. Cieślińska and E. Kostyra, "Polymorphism of bovine beta-casein and its potential effect on human health," *J Appl Genet,* vol. 48, 2007, p. 189–98.

90. C.N. McLachlan, "Beta-casein A1, ischaemic heart disease mortality, and other illnesses," *Med hypotheses,* vol. 56, 2001, p. 262–72; M. Laugesen and R. Elliot, "Ischaemic heart disease, type 1 diabetes, and cow milk A1 beta-casein," *N Z Med J,* vol. 116, 2003, p. 1–19.

91. G. Kontopidis, C. Holt and L. Sawyer, "Invited review: Beta-lactoglobulin: Binding properties, structure, and function," *J Dairy Sci,* vol. 87, 2004, p. 785–96; R.G. Jensen, "The composition of bovine milk lipids: January 1995 to December 2000," *J Dairy Sci,* vol. 85, 2002, p. 295–350.

92. J.W. Anderson, B.M. Johnstone and D.T. Remley, "Breast-feeding and cognitive development: A meta-analysis," *Am J Clin Nutr,* vol. 70, 1999, p. 525–35.

93. L. Shack-Nielsen and K.F. Michaelsen, "Advances in our understanding of the biology of human milk and its effects on the offspring," *J Nutrition,* vol. 137, 2007, p. 503S–10S.

94. B.C. Melnik, "Milk: The promoter of chronic Western diseases," *Med Hypotheses,* vol. 72, 2009, p. 631–39.

95. J.W. Rich-Edwards, D. Ganmaa, M.N. Pollak et al., "Milk consumption and the prepubertal somatotropic axis," *Nutr J,* vol. 6, 2007, p. 28; A. Larnkjaer, H.K. Ingstrup, L. Schack-Nielsen et al., "Early programming of the IGF-I axis: Negative association between IGF-I in infancy and late adolescence in a 17-year longitudinal follow-up study of healthy subjects," *Growth Horm IGF Res,* vol. 19, 2009, p. 82–86.

96. A. Denley, L.J. Cosgrove, G.W. Booker et al., "Molecular interactions of the IGF system," *Cytokine Growth Factor Rev 2005,* vol. 16, 2005, p. 421–39.

97. A. Denley, J.C. Wallace, L.J. Cosgrove et al., "The insulin receptor isoform exon 11-(IR-A) in cancer and other diseases: A review," *Horm Metab Res,* vol. 35, 2003, p. 778–85.

98. G. Furstenberger and H.J. Senn, "Insulin-like growth factors and cancer," *Lancet,* vol. 3, 2002, p. 298–302.

99. M. Gaard, S. Tretli and E.B. Loken, "Dietary fat and the risk of breast cancer: A prospective study of 25,892 Norwegian Women," *Int J Cancer,* vol. 63, 1995, p. 13–17.

100. Writing Group for the Women's Health Initiative Investigators, "Risks and benefits of estrogen plus progestin in healthy postmenopausal women," *JAMA,* vol. 288, 2002, p. 321–33.

101. S. Demers, *Hormones au féminin,* Montréal, Les Éditions de l'Homme, 2008, 259 p.

102. G.L. Francis, F.M. Upton, F.J. Ballard et al., "Insulin-like growth factors 1 and 2 in bovine colostrum: Sequences and biological activities compared with those of a potent truncated form," *Biochem J,* vol. 251, 1988, p. 95–103.

103. M.D. Holmes, M.N. Pollak, W.C. Willett et al., "Dietary correlates of plasma insulin-like growth factor-1 and insulin-like growth factor binding protein 3 concentrations," *Cancer Epidemiol Biomarkers Prev,* vol. 11, 2002, p. 852–61; I.S. Rogers, D. Gunnell, P.M. Emmett et al., "Cross-sectional associations of diet and insulin-like growth factor levels in 7-to-8-year-old children," *Cancer Epidemiol Biomarkers Prev,* vol. 14, 2005, p. 204–12.

104. E.M. Ostman, H.G.M. Liljeberg Elmstahl and I.M.E. Bjorck, "Inconsistency between glycemic and insulinemic responses to regular and fermented milk products," *Am J Clin Nutr,* vol. 74, 2001, p. 96–100.

105. G. Hoyt, M.S. Hickey and L. Cordain, "Dissociation of the glycaemic and insulinaemic responses to whole and skimmed milk," *Br J Nutr,* vol. 93, 2005, p. 175–77.

106. M.C. Gannon, F.Q. Nuttal, P.A. Krezowski et al., "The serum insulin and plasma glucose responses to milk and fruit in type 2 (non-insulin-dependent) diabetic patients," *Diabetologica,* vol. 29, 1986, p. 784–91.

107. S. Holt, J. Brand Miller and p. Petocz, "An insulin index of foods: The insulin demand generated by 1000-kj portions of common foods," *Am J Clin Nutr,* vol. 66, 1997, p. 1264–76.

108. B.C. Melnik, "Milk: The promoter of chronic Western diseases," *Med Hypotheses,* vol. 72, 2009, p. 631–39.

109. A. Larnkjaer, H.K. Ingstrup, L. Schack-Nielsen et al., "Early programming of the IGF-I axis: Negative association between IGF-I in infancy and late adolescence in a 17-year longitudinal follow-up study of healthy subjects," *Growth Horm IGF Res,* vol. 19, 2009, p. 82–86.
110. B.C. Melnik, "Milk: The promoter of chronic Western diseases," *Med Hypotheses,* vol. 72, 2009, p. 631–39.
111. S. Holt, J. Brand Miller and P. Petocz, "An insulin index of foods: The insulin demand generated by 1000-kj portions of common foods," *Am J Clin Nutr,* vol. 66, 1997, p. 1264–76.
112. K. Dahl-Jorgensen, G. Joner and K.F. Hanssen, "Relationship between cows' milk consumption and incidence of IDDM in childhood," *Diabetes Care,* vol. 14, 1991, p. 1081–83.
113. R.E. LaPorte, N. Tajima, H.K. Akerblom et al., "Geographic differences in the risk of insulin-dependent diabetes mellitus: The importance of registries," *Diabetes Care,* vol. 8, Suppl. 1, 1985, p. 101–07.
114. The Diamond Project Group, "Incidence and trends of childhood type 1 diabetes worldwide 1990-1999," *J Compilation,* vol. 23, 2006, p. 857–66.
115. The Diamond Project Group, "Incidence and trends of childhood type 1 diabetes worldwide 1990–1999," *J Compilation,* vol. 23, 2006, p. 857–66.
116. B.C. Melnik, "Milk: The promoter of chronic Western diseases," *Med Hypotheses,* vol. 72, 2009, p. 631–39.
117. Gale EAM, "The rise of childhood type 1 diabetes in the 20th century," *Diabetes,* vol. 51, 2002, p. 3353–61.
118. The Diamond Project Group, "Incidence and trends of childhood type 1 diabetes worldwide 1990-1999," *J Compilation,* vol. 23, 2006, p. 857–66.
119. T.C. Campbell and T.M. Campbell, *Le Rapport Campbell. Révélations stupéfiantes sur les liens entre L'Alimentation et la santé à long terme,* Outremont, Éditions Ariane, 2008, 488 p.; C. Kousmine, *Sauvez votre corps,* Paris, Éditions J'ai lu, 1987, 629 p.
120. C. Kousmine, *Sauvez votre corps,* Paris, Editions J'ai lu, 1987, 629 p.; R.L. Hostettler-Allen, L. Tappy and J.W. Blum, "Insulin resistance, hyperglycemia, and glucosuria in intensively milk-fed calves," *J Anim Sci,* vol. 72, 1994, p. 160–73.
121. R.L. Hostettler-Allen, L. Tappy and J.W. Blum, "Insulin resistance hyperglycemia, and glucosuria in intensively milk-fed calves," *J Anim Sci,* vol. 72, 1994, p. 160–173.
122. R. Wolter, *Alimentation de la vache laitière,* 3e édition, Paris, Édition La France agricole, 1997, 264 p.
123. R.P. Heaney, "Bone as the calcium nutrient reserve," in C.M. Weaver, R.P. Heaney (dir.), *Calcium in human health,* Totowa, Human Press Inc.

2006, p. 7–12; K. Rafferty and R.P. Heaney, "Nutrient effects on the calcium economy: Emphasizing the potassium controversy," *J Nutr,* vol. 138, 2008, p. 166S–171S.

124. J. Brockie, "Exercise for women in the early postmenopausal years," *J Br Menopause Soc,* vol. 12, 2006, p. 126–27; A. Guadalupe-Grau, T. Fuentes, B. Guerra et al., "Exercise and bone mass in adults," *Sports Med,* vol. 39, 2009, p. 439–68.

125. J. Compston, "Clinical and therapeutic aspects of osteoporosis," *Eur J Radiol,* vol. 71, 2009, p. 388–91.

126. P. Haentjens, J. Magaziner, C.S. Colon-Emeric et al., "Meta-analysis: Excess mortality after hip fracture among older women and men," *Ann Intern Med,* vol. 152, 2010, p. 380–90.

127. B.J. Abelow, T.R. Holford and K.L. Insogna, "Cross-cultural association between dietary animal protein and hip fracture: A hypothesis," *Calcif Tissue Int,* vol. 50, 1992, p. 14–18.

128. D. Feskanich, W.C. Willet, M.J. Stampfer et al., "Milk, dietary calcium, and bone fractures in women: A 12-year prospective study," *Am J Public Health,* vol. 87, 1997, p. 992–97; K. Michaelsson, H. Melhus, R. Bellocco et al., "Dietary calcium and vitamin D in relation to osteoporotic fracture risk," *Bone,* vol. 32, 2003, p. 694–03.

129. A. Bischoff-Ferrari, B. Dawson-Hughes, J.A. Baron et al., "Calcium intake and hip fracture risk in men and women: A meta-analysis of prospective cohort studies and randomized controlled trials," *Am J Clin Nutr,* vol. 86, 2007, p. 1780–90; J.A. Kanis, H. Johansson, A. Oden et al., "A meta-analysis of milk intake and fracture risk: Low utility for case finding," *Osteoporos Int,* vol. 16, 2005, p. 799–04.

130. C.S. Johnston, S.L. Tjonn, P.D. Swan et al., "Low-carbohydrate, high-protein diets that restrict potassium-rich fruits and vegetables promote calciuria," *Osteoporos Int,* vol. 17, 2006, p. 1820–21.

131. J. Vormann and T. Remer, "Dietary, metabolic, physiologic, and disease related aspects of acid-base balance: Foreword to the contributions of the second international acid-base symposium," *J Nutr,* vol. 138, 2008, p. 413S–14S.

132. S. Berkemeyer, J. Vormann, A.L.B. Gunther et al., "Renal net acid excretion capacity is comparable in repubescence, adolescence, and young adulthood but falls with aging," JAGS, vol. 56, 2008, p. 1442–48; B. Dawson-Hughes, S.S. Harris, N.J. Palermo et al., "Treatment with potassium bicarbonate lowers calcium excretion and bone resorption in older men and women," *J Clin Endocrinol Metab,* vol. 94, 2009, p. 96–102.

133. Ibid.

134. L.A. Frassetto and C. Hsu, "Metabolic acidosis and progression of chronic kidney disease," *J Am Soc Nephrol,* vol. 20, 2009, p. 1869–70; I. Brito-Ashurst, M. Varagunam, M.J. Raferty et al., "Bicarbonate supplementation slows progression of CKD and improves nutritional status," *J Am Soc Nephrol,* vol. 20, 2009, p. 2075–84.

135. M. Gaard, S. Tretli and E.B. Loken, "Dietary fat and the risk of breast cancer: A prospective study of 25,892 Norwegian women," *Int J Cancer,* vol. 63, 1995, p. 13–17; J. Green and C.R. Kleeman, "Role of bone in regulation of systemic acid-base balance," *Kidney Int,* vol. 39, 1991, p. 9–26.

136. H.M. Macdonald, A.J. Black, L. Aucott et al., "Effect of potassium citrate supplementation or increased fruit and vegetable intake on bone metabolism in healthy postmenopausal women: A randomized controlled trial," *Am J Clin Nutr,* vol. 88, 2008, p. 465–74; S.A. New, C. Bolton-Smith, D.A. Grubb et al., "Nutritional influences on bone mineral density: A cross-sectional study in menopausal women," *Am J Clin Nutr,* vol. 65, 1997, p. 1831–39; H.M. Macdonald, S.A. New, M.H. Golden et al., "Nutritional associations with bone loss during the menopausal transition: Evidence of a beneficial effect of calcium, alcohol, and fruit and vegetable nutrients and of a detrimental effect of fatty acids," *Am J Clin Nutr,* vol. 79, 2004, p. 155–65.

137. L.A. Frassetto, R.C. Morris, Jr., E. Sellmeyer et al., "Adverse effects of sodium chloride on bone in the aging human population resulting from habitual consumption of typical American diets," *J Nutr,* vol. 138, 2008, p. 419S–22S.

138. L.A. Frassetto, R.C. Morris, Jr., E. Sellmeyer et al., "Adverse effects of sodium chloride on bone in the aging human population resulting from habitual consumption of typical American diets," *J Nutr,* vol. 138, 2008, p. 419S–22S; P. Frings-Meuthen, N. Baecker and M. Heer, "Low-grade metabolic acidosis may be the cause of sodium chloride-induced exaggerated bone resorption," *J Bone Miner Res,* vol. 23, 2008, p. 517–24.

139. Report of a Joint FAO/WHO Expert Consultation, "Human vitamin and mineral requirements," September 1998, Bangkok, Thailand. Available at: ftp://ftp.fao.org/es/esn/nutrition/Vitrni/vitrni.html (accessed October 24, 2008).

140. U.S. Department of Agriculture, "Agricultural Research Service, USDA Nutrient Data Laboratory, 2007. USDA National Nutrient Database for Standard Reference," Release 20. Available at: www.ars.usda.gov/ nutrientdata (accessed October 24, 2008); N.D. Barnard, A.R. Scialli, G. Truner-McGrievy et al., "The effects of a low-fat, plant-based dietary intervention on body weight, metabolism, and insulin sensitivity," *Am J Med,* vol. 118, 2005, p. 991–97.

141. I. Jennifer, R.D. Keller, J. Amy et al., "The consumer cost of calcium from food and supplements," *J Am Diet Assoc,* vol. 102, 2002, p. 1669–71; U.S. Barzel and L.K. Massey, "Excess dietary protein can adversely affect bone," *J Nutr,* vol. 128, 1998, p. 1051–53.

142. C.M. Weaver, W.R. Proulx and R. Heaney, "Choices for achieving adequate dietary calcium with a vegetarian diet," *Am J Clin Nutr,* vol. 70 (suppl.), 1999, p. 543S–48S; A.J. Lanou, "Should dairy be recommended as part of a healthy vegetarian diet? Counterpoint," *Am J Clin Nutr,* vol. 89 (suppl.), 2009, p. 1638S–42S.

143. I. Seiquer, M. Mesias, A.M. Hoyos et al., "A Mediterranean dietary style improves calcium utilization in healthy male adolescents," *J Am Coll Nutr,* vol. 27, 2008, p. 454–62.

144. S.A. New, S.P. Robins, M.K. Campbell et al., "Dietary influences on bone mass and bone metabolism: Further evidence of a positive link between fruit and vegetable consumption and bone health?" *Am J Clin Nutr,* vol. 71, 2000, p. 142–51; C.J. Prynne, G.D. Mishra, M.A. O'Connel et al., "Fruit and vegetable intake and bone mineral status: A cross-sectional study in 5 age and sex cohorts," *Am J Clin Nutr,* vol. 83, 2006, p. 1420–28.

145. www.passeportsante.net; I. Jennifer, R.D. Keller, J. Amy et al., "The consumer cost of calcium from food and supplements," *J Am Diet Assoc,* vol. 102, 2002, p. 1669–71; A.J. Lanou, "Should dairy be recommended as part of a healthy vegetarian diet? Counterpoint," *Am J Clin Nutr,* vol. 89 (suppl.), 2009, p. 1638S–42S; C.M. Weaver and K.L. Plawecki, "Dietary calcium: Adequacy of a vegetarian diet," *Am J Clin Nutr,* vol. 59 (suppl.), 1994, p. 1238S–41S.

146. C.D. Hunt and L.K. Johnson, "Calcium requirements: New estimations for men and women by cross-sectional statistical analyses of calcium balance data from metabolic studies," *Am J Clin Nutr,* vol. 86, 2007, p. 1054–63.

147. R.P. Heaney, "Calcium," in J.P. Bilezikian, L.G. Raiz and G.A. Rodan (dir.), *Principles of bone biology,* San Diego (CA), Academic, 1996, p. 1007–18.

148. "Guide alimentaire canadien," www.hc-sc.gc.ca/fr.

149. C.D. Hunt and L.K. Johnson, "Calcium requirements: New estimations for men and women by cross-sectional statistical analyses of calcium balance data from metabolic studies," *Am J Clin Nutr,* vol. 86, 2007, p. 1054–63.

150. A.C. Looker and M.E. Mussolino, "Serum 25-hydroxyvitamin D and hip fracture risk in older U.S. white adults," *J Bone Miner Res,* vol. 23, 2008, p. 143–50.

151. K.L. Tucker, M.T. Hannan, H. Chen et al., "Potassium, magnesium, and fruit and vegetable intake are associated with greater bone mineral density in elderly men and women," *Am J Clin Nutr,* vol. 69, 1999, p. 726–36.

152. J.A. Simon and E.S. Hudes, "Relation of ascorbic acid to bone mineral density and self-reported fractures among US adults," *Am J Epidemiol,* vol. 154, 2001, p. 427–33; K.L. Tucker, "Osteoporosis Prevention and Nutrition," *Current Osteoporosis Reports,* vol. 7, 2009, p. 111–17.

153. D. Feskanich, P. Weber, W.C. Willett et al., "Vitamin K intake and hip fractures in women: A prospective study," *Am J Clin Nutr,* vol. 69, 1999, p. 74–79.

154. S. Sahni, M.T. Hannan, J. Blumberg et al., "Protective effect of total carotenoid and lycopene intake on the risk of hip fracture: A 17-year follow-up from the Framingham Osteoporosis Study," *J Bone Miner Res,* vol. 24, 2009, p. 1086–94.

155. K.L. Tucker, "Osteoporosis Prevention and Nutrition," *Current Osteoporosis Reports,* vol. 7, 2009, p. 111–17.

156. Ibid.

157. T. Lloyd, V.M. Chinchilli, N. Johnson-Rollings et al., "Adult female hip bone density reflects teenage sports-exercise patterns but not teenage calcium intake," *Pediatrics,* vol. 106, 2000, p. 40–44; W. Kemmier, S. von Stengel, K. Engelke et al., "Exercise effects on bone mineral density, falls, coronary risk factors, and health care costs in older women: The randomized controlled senior fitness and prevention (SEFIP) study," *Arch Intern Med,* vol. 170, 2010, p. 179–85.

158. E. Wynn, M.A. Krieg, J.M. Aeschlimann, P. Burckhardt, "Alkaline mineral water lowers bone resorption even in calcium sufficiency: Alkaline mineral water and bone metabolism," *Bone,* vol. 44, 2009, p. 120–24.

159. P. Meunier, C. Jenvrin, F. Munoz et al., "Consumption of a high calcium mineral water lowers biochemical indices of bone remodelling in postmenopausal women with low calcium intake," *Osteoporos Int,* vol. 16, 2005, p. 1203–09; J. Guillemant, L. Huyen-Tran, C. Accarie et al., "Mineral water as a source of dietary calcium: Acute effects on parathyroid function and bone resorption in young men," *Am J Clin Nutr,* vol. 71, 2000, p. 999–1002.

160. L.C. Maillard, "Action des acides amines sur des sucres: Formation des mélanoides par voie méthodique," *C R Acad Sci,* vol. 154, 1912, p. 66–68.

161. Van Nguyen C, "Toxicity of the AGEs generated from the Maillard reaction: On the relationship of food-AGEs and biological-AGEs," *Mol Nutr Food Res,* vol. 50, 2006, p. 1140–49; S.R. Thorpe et J.W. Baynes, "Maillard reaction products in tissue proteins: New products and new perspectives," *Amino Acids,* vol. 25, 2003, p. 275–81.

162. C. Van Nguyen, "Toxicity of the AGEs generated from the Maillard reaction: On the relationship of food-AGEs and biological-AGEs," *Mol Nutr Food Res,* vol. 50, 2006, p. 1140–49; M.A. Saraiva, C.M. Borges and M.H. Florencio, "Non-enzymatic model glycation reactions: A comprehensive

study of the reactivity of a modified arginine with aldehydic and diketonic dicarbonyl compounds by electrospray mass spectrometry," *J Mass Spectrom,* 41, 2006, p. 755–70; P. Pouillart, H. Mauprivez, L. Ait-Ameur et al., "Strategy for the study of the health impact of dietary Maillard products in clinical studies: The example of the ICARE clinical study on healthy adults," *Ann NY Acad Sci,* vol. 1126, 2008, p. 173–76; H. Vlassara, "Advanced glycation in health and disease: Role of the modern environment," *Ann NY Acad Sci,* vol. 1043, 2005, p. 452–60.

163. J. Uribarri, S. Woodruff, S. Goodman et al., "Advanced glycation end products in foods and a practical guide to their reduction in the diet," *Am Diet Ass,* vol. 110, 2010, p. 912–16.

164. C. Van Nguyen, "Toxicity of the AGEs generated from the Maillard reaction: On the relationship of food-AGEs and biological-AGEs," *Mol Nutr Food Res,* vol. 50, 2006, p. 1140–49; S.R. Thorpe et J.W. Baynes, "Maillard reaction products in tissue proteins: New products and new perspectives," *Amino Acids,* vol. 25, 2003, p. 275–81.

165. T. Chavakis, A. Bierhaus and P.P. Nawroth, "RAGE (receptor for advanced glycation end products): A central player in the inflammatory response," *Microbes Infect,* vol. 6, 2004, p. 1219-25; R. Ramasamy, S.J. Vannucci, S.S. Yan et al., "Advanced glycation end products and RAGE: A common thread in aging, diabetes, neurodegeneration, and inflammation," *Glycobiology,* vol. 15, 2005, p. 16R–28R.

166. A. Xanthis, A. Hatzitolios, G. Koliakos et al., "Advanced glycosylation end products and nutrition: A possible relation with diabetic atherosclerosis and how to prevent it," *J Food Sci,* vol. 72, 2007, p. R125–29.

167. S. Bengmark, "Advanced glycation and lipoxidation end products— amplifiers of inflammation: The role of food," *J Parenter Enteral Nutr,* vol. 31, 2007, p. 430–40.

168. H. Vlassara, J. Cai, J. Crandall et al., "Inflammatory mediators are induced by dietary glycotoxins, a major risk factor for diabetic angiopathy," *Proc Natl Acad Sci USA,* vol. 99, 2002, p. 15596–601; M. Peppa, J. Uribarri, W. Cai et al., "Glyoxidation and inflammation in renal failure patients," *Am J Kidney Dis,* vol. 43, 2004, p. 690–95.

169. R. Weindruch, "The retardation of aging by caloric restriction: Studies in rodents and primates," *Toxicol Pathol,* vol. 24, 1996, p. 742–45; J. Couzin, "Low-calorie diets may slow monkeys' aging," *Science,* vol. 282, 1998, p. 1018.

170. H. Vlassara, "Advanced glycation in health and disease: Role of the modern environment," *Ann NY Acad. Sci.,* vol. 1043, 2005, p. 452–60; W. Cai, J.C. He, L. Zhu et al., "Reduced oxidant stress and extended lifespan in mice exposed to a low glycotoxin diet: Association with increased AGER1 expression," *Am J Pathol,* vol. 170, 2007, p. 1893–1902.

171. H. Vlassara and G. Striker, "Glycotoxins in the diet promote diabetes and diabetic complications," *Curr DiabRep,* vol. 7, 2007, p. 235–41; J. Uribarri, M. Peppa, W. Cai et al., "Restriction of dietary glycotoxins markedly reduces AGE toxins in renal failure patients," *J Am Soc Nephrol,* vol. 14, 2003, p. 728–31.

172. J. Uribarri, W. Cai, M. Peppa et al., "Circulating glycotoxins and dietary advanced glycation endproducts: Two links to inflammatory response, oxidative stress, and aging," *J Gerontol A Bio Sci Med Sci,* vol. 62, 2007, p. 427–33; I. Birlouez-Aragon, F. Morales, V. Fogliano et al., "The health and technological implications of a better control of neoformed contaminants by the food industry," *Pathol Biol* (Paris), vol. 58, 2010, p. 232–38.

173. T. Neade and J. Uribarri, "Diet, inflammation, and chronic kidney disease: Getting to the heart of the matter," *Semin Dial,* vol. 21, 2008, p. 331–37.

174. J. Uribarri, W. Cai, O. Sandu et al., "Diet-derived advanced glycation end products are major contributors to the body's AGE pool and induce inflammation in healthy subjects," *Ann NY Acad Sci,* vol. 1043, 2005, p. 461–66.

175. Ibid.

176. T. Korchinsky, C.J. He, T. Mitsuhashi et al., "Orally absorbed reactive glycation products (glycotoxins): An environmental risk factor in diabetic nephropathy," *Proc Natl Acad Sci U S A,* vol. 94, 1997, p. 6474–79.

177. H. Vlassara, J. Uribarri, L. Ferrucci et al., "Identifying advanced glycation end products as a major source of oxidants in aging: Implications for the management and/or prevention of reduced renal function in elderly persons," *Semin Nephrol,* vol. 29, 2009, p. 594–603.

178. M. Peppa and S.A. Raptis, "Advanced glycation end products and cardiovascular disease," *Curr Diabetes Rev,* vol. 4, 2008, p. 92–100; H. Vlassara, J. Uribarri, W. Cai et al., "Advanced glycation end product homeostasis: Exogenous oxidants and innate defenses," *Ann NY Acad Sci,* vol. 1126, 2008, p. 46–52.

179. C. Van Nguyen, "Toxicity of the AGEs generated from the Maillard reaction: On the relationship of food-AGEs and biological-AGEs," *Mol Nutr Food Res,* vol. 50, 2006, p. 1140–49.

180. H. Vlassara, J. Uribarri, W. Cai et al., "Advanced glycation end product homeostasis: Exogenous oxidants and innate defenses," *Ann NY Acad Sci,* vol. 1126, 2008, p. 46–52; B.S. Szwergold, S.K. Howell and P.J. Beisswenger, "Human fructosamine-3-kinase: Purification, sequencing, substrate specificity, and evidence of activity in vivo," *Diabetes,* vol. 50, 2001, p. 2139–47.

181. W. Cai, J.C. He, L. Zhu et al., "Oral glycotoxins determine the effects of calorie restriction on oxidant stress, age-related diseases, and lifespan," *Am J Pathol,* vol. 173, 2008, p. 327–35; H. Vlassara, W. Cai, S. Goodman et al., "Protection against loss of innate defenses in adulthood by low advanced glycation end products (AGE) intake: Role of the anti-inflammatory AGE receptor-1," *J Clin Endocrinol Metab,* vol. 94, 2009, p. 4483–91.

182. H. Vlassara, W. Cai, S. Goodman et al., "Protection against loss of innate defences in adulthood by low advanced glycation end products (AGE) intake: Role of the antiinflammatory AGE receptor-1," *J Clin Endocrinol Metab,* vol. 94, 2009, p. 4483–91; M. Torreggiani, H. Liu, J. Wu et al., "Advanced glycation end product receptor-1 transgenic mice are resistant to inflammation, oxidative stress, and post-injury intimal hyperplasia," *Am J Pathol,* vol. 175, 2009, p. 1722.

183. H. Vlassara, J. Uribarri, W. Cai et al., "Advanced glycation end product homeostasis: Exogenous oxidants and innate defenses," *Ann NY Acad Sci,* vol. 1126, 2008, p. 46–52.

184. D. Aronson, "Cross-linking of glycated collagen in the pathogenesis of arterial and myocardial stiffening of aging and diabetes," *J Hypertens,* vol. 21, 2003, p. 3–12.

185. S. Bengmark, "Advanced glycation and lipoxidation end products-amplifiers of inflammation: The role of food," *J Parenter Enteral Nutr,* vol. 31, 2007, p. 430–40.

186. Ibid.

187. T. Goldberg, W. Cai, M. Peppa et al., "Advanced glycoxidation end products in commonly consumed foods," *J Am Diet Assoc,* vol. 104, 2004, p. 1287–91.

188. S. Bengmark, "Advanced glycation and lipoxidation end products—amplifiers of inflammation: The role of food," *J Parenter Enteral Nutr,* vol. 31, 2007, p. 430–40.

189. T. Goldberg, W. Cai, M. Peppa et al., "Advanced glycoxidation end products in commonly consumed foods," *J Am Diet Assoc,* vol. 104, 2004, p. 1287–91.

190. A. Xanthis, A. Hatzitolios, G. Koliakos et al., "Advanced glycosylation end products and nutrition: A possible relation with diabetic atherosclerosis and how to prevent it," *J Food Sci,* vol. 72, 2007, p. R125–29.

191. J. Uribarri, S. Wooddruff, S. Goodman et al., "Advanced glycation end products in foods and a practical guide to their reduction in the diet," *Am Diet Ass,* vol. 110, 2010, p. 912–16.

192. Ibid.

193. Ibid.

194. I. Birlouez-Aragon, F. Morales, V. Fogliano et al., "The health and technological implications of a better control of neoformed contaminants by the food industry," *Pathol Biol* (Paris), vol. 58, 2010, p. 232–38.

195. M.I. Sabri and P.S. Spencer, "How does acrylamide perturb axon transport and induce nerve fiber degeneration? Commentary on forum position paper," *Neurotoxicology,* vol. 23, 2002, p. 259–63.

196. E. Tareke, p. Rydberg, p. Karlsson et al., "Analysis of acrylamide, a carcinogen formed in heated foodstuffs," *J Agric Food Chem,* vol. 50, 2002, p. 4998–5006.

197. G. Weiss, "Acrylamide in Food: Uncharted Territory," *Science,* vol. 297, 2002, p. 27.

198. D.S. Mottram, B.L. Wedzicha and A.T. Dodson, "Food chemistry: Acrylamide is formed in the Maillard reaction," *Nature,* vol. 419, 2002, p. 448–49.

199. W. Ahmad, L. Li and Y. Deng, "Identification of AGE-precursors and AGE formation in glycation-induced BSA peptides," *BMB Rep,* vol. 41, 2008, p. 516–22; Y.L. Lai, S. Aoyama, R. Nagai et al., "Inhibition of L-arginine metabolizing enzymes by L-arginine-derived advanced glycation end products," *J Clin Biochem Nutr,* vol. 46, 2010, p. 177–85.

200. M. Friedman and C.E. Levin, "Review of methods for the reduction of dietary content and toxicity of acrylamide," *J Agric Food Chem,* vol. 56, 2008, p. 6113–40.

201. Ibid.

202. Ibid.

203. Ibid.

204. R. Nishigaki, T. Watanabe, T. Kajimoto et al., "Isolation and identification of a novel aromatic amine mutagen produced by the Maillard reaction," *Chem Res Toxicol,* vol. 22, 2009, p. 1588–93.

205. R. Abe et S. Yamagishi, "AGE-RAGE system and carcinogenesis," *Curr Pharm Des,* vol. 15, 2008, p. 940–45.

206. Ibid.

207. C. Kousmine, *Sauvez votre corps,* Paris, Éditions J'ai lu, 1987, 629 p.

208. J. Uribarri, W. Cai, M. Peppa et al., "Circulating glycotoxins and dietary advanced glycation endproducts: Two links to inflammatory response, oxidative stress, and aging," *J Gerontol A Bio Sci Med Sci,* vol. 62, 2007, p. 427–33; I. Birlouez-Aragon, F. Morales, V. Fogliano et al., "The health and technological implications of a better control of neoformed contaminants by the food industry," *Pathol Biol* (Paris), vol. 58, 2010, p. 232–38.

209. T.H. Parliament, "Comparison of thermal and microwave mediated Maillard reactions," *Dev-Food-Sci,* vol.32, 1993, Amsterdam: Elsevier Scientific Publications, p. 657–62.

210. Ibid.

5 BASIC PRINCIPLES OF THE HYPOTOXIC DIET

1. K. Sakai, L.A. Frassetto, M. Schloetter et al., "Metabolic and physiologic improvements from consuming a paleolithic, hunter-gatherer type diet," *Eur J Clin Nutr,* vol. 63, 2009, p. 947–55.

2. I. Birlouez-Aragon, F. Morales, V. Fogliano et al., "The health and technological implications of a better control of neoformed contaminants by the food industry," *Pathol Biol* (Paris), vol. 58, 2010, p. 232-38.

3. E. Capuano, A. Ferrigno, I. Acampa et al., "Characterization of the Maillard reaction in bread crisp," *Eur Food Res Technol,* vol. 228, 2008, p. 311–19.

4. W. Ahmad, L. Li and Y. Deng, "Identification of AGE-precursors and AGE formation in glycation-induced BSA peptides," *BMB Rep,* vol. 41, 2008, p. 516–22.

5. K. Nakano, T. Suzuki, T. Hayakawa et al., "Organ and cellular localization of asparagine synthetase in rice plants," *Plant Cell Physiol,* vol. 41, 2000, p. 874–80.

6. Y. Kezuka, T. Itagaki, R. Satoh et al., "Purification, crystallization and preliminary X-ray analysis of a deletion mutant of a major buckwheat allergen," *Acta Crystallogr Sect F Struct Biol Cryst Commun,* vol. 65, 2009, p. 1267–70.

7. II. Zielinski, A. Michalska, M. Amigo-Benavent et al., "Changes in protein quality and antioxidant properties of buckwheat seeds and groats induced by roasting," *J Agric Food Chem,* vol. 57, 2009, p. 4771–76.

8. K. Sakai, S. Kino, M. Takeuchi et al., "Analysis of antioxydant activities in vegetable oils and fat soluble vitamins and biofactors by the PAO-SO method," *Methods Mol Biol,* vol. 594, 2010, p. 241–50.

9. J. Uribarri, S. Woodruff, S. Goodman et al., "Advanced glycation end products in foods and a practical guide to their reduction in the diet," *Am Diet Ass,* vol. 110, 2010, p. 912–16.

6 MAINTAINING A PROPER PHYSIOLOGICAL BALANCE: PRODUCTS, PRINCIPLES AND INFORMATION

1. M. Messina and A.H. Wu, "Perspectives on the soy-breast cancer relation," *Am J Clin Nutr,* vol. 89 (suppl.), 2009, p. 1673s–79s.

2. B.J. Trock, L. Hilakivi-Clarke and R. Clarke, "Meta-analysis of soy intake and breast cancer risk," *J Natl Cancer Inst,* vol. 98, 2006, p. 459–71.

3. A. Jacobs, U. Wegewitz, C. Sommerfeld et al., "Efficacy of isoflavones in relieving vasomotor menopausal symptoms: A systematic review," *Mol Nutr Food Res,* vol. 53, 2009, p. 1084–97.

4. M. Messina, W. McCaskill-Stevens and J.W. Lampe, "Addressing the soy and breast cancer relationship: Review, commentary, and workshop proceedings," *J Natl Cancer Inst,* vol. 98, 2006, p. 1275–84.

5. D. Rieu, A. Bocquet, J.-L. Bresson et al., "Phyto-estrogènes et aliments à base de soja chez le nourrisson et l'enfant: la prudence est de mise," *Arch pediatr,* vol. 13, 2006, p. 1091–93.

6. Y. Cao, A.M. Calafat, D.R. Doerge et al., "Isoflavones in urine, saliva and blood of infants: Data from a pilot study on the estrogenic activity of soy formula," *J Expo Sci Environ Epidemiol,* vol. 19, 2009, p. 223–34.

7. W.Z. Zhang, W.M. Cui, X. Zhang et al., "Subchronic toxicity study on soy isoflavones in rats," *Biomedical and Environmental Sciences,* vol. 22, 2009, p. 259–64; L. Guan, Y. Huang and Z. Chen, "Developmental and reproductive toxicity of soybean isoflavones to immature SD rats," *Biomed Environ Sci,* vol. 21, 2008, p. 197–204; L. Pan, X. Xia, Y. Feng et al., "Exposure to the phytoestrogen daidzein attenuates apomorphine-induced penile erection concomitant with plasma testosterone level reduction in dose- and time-related manner in adults rats," *Urology,* vol. 70, 2007, p. 613–17; D.J. Kim, S.H. Seok, M.W. Baek et al., "Developmental toxicity and brain aromatase induction by high genistein concentrations in zebrafish embryos," *Toxicol Mech Methods,* vol. 19, 2009, p. 251–56; S. Basak, D. Pookot, E. Noonan et al., "Genistein down-regulates androgen receptor by modulating HDAC6-Hsp90 chaperone function," *Mol Cancer Ther,* vol. 7, 2008, p. 3195–202; J. D. Sherrill, M. Sparks, J. Dennis et al., "Developmental exposures of male rats to soy isoflavones impact Leydig cell differentiation," *Biol Reprod,* vol. 83, 2010, p. 488–501.

8. A. Faqi, W. Johnson, R. Morrissey et al., "Reproductive toxicity assessment of chronic dietary exposure to soy isoflavones in male rats," *Reprod Toxicol,* vol. 18, 2004, p. 605–11; T.M. Badger, J.M. Gilchrist, R.T. Pivik et al., "The health implications of soy infant formula," *Am J Clin Nutr,* vol. 89 (suppl.), 2009, p. 1668S–1672.

9. K.D. Hancock, E.S. Coleman, Y.X. Tao et al., "Genistein decreases androgen biosynthesis in rat Leydig cells by interference with luteinizing hormone dependent signalling," *Toxicol Lett,* vol. 184, 2009, p. 169–75.

10. D.J. Kim, S.H. Seok, M.W. Baek et al., "Developmental toxicity and brain aromatase induction by high genistein concentrations in zebrafish embryos," *Toxicol Mech Methods,* vol. 19, 2009, p. 251–56.

11. E.N. Pearce and L.E. Braverman, "Environmental pollutants and the thyroid," *Best Pract Res Clin Endocrinol Metab,* vol. 23, 2009, p. 801–13.

12. R. Hampl, D. Ostatnikova, P. Celec et al., "Short-term effect of soy consumption on thyroid hormone levels and correlation with phytoestrogen level in healthy subjects," *Endocr Regul,* vol. 42, 2008, p. 53–61.

13. M. Messina and G. Redmond, "Effects of soy protein and soybean isoflavones on thyroid function in healthy adults and hypothyroid patients: A review of the relevant literature," *Thyroid,* vol. 16, 2006, p. 249–58

14. P. Burckhardt, "The effects of the alkali load of mineral water on bone metabolism: Interventional studies," *J Nutr,* vol. 138, 2008, p. 435s–37s.

15. H. Bhmer, H. Miller and K.L. Resch, "Calcium supplementation with calcium rich mineral waters: A systemic review and meta-analysis of its bioavailability," *Osteoporos Int,* vol. 11, 2000, p. 938–43.

16. E. Wynn, M.A. Krieg, J.M. Aeschlimann, p. Burckhardt, "Alkaline mineral water lowers bone resorption even in calcium sufficiency: Alkaline mineral water and bone metabolism," *Bone,* vol. 44, 2009, p. 120–24; P. Burckhardt, "The effects of the alkali load of mineral water on bone metabolism: Interventional studies," *J Nutr,* vol. 138, 2008, p. 435s–37s.

17. E. Wynn, E. Raetz and p. Burckhardt, "The composition of mineral waters sourced from Europe and North America in respect to bone health: Composition of mineral water optimal for bone," *British Journal of Nutrition,* vol. 101, 2009, p. 1195–199.

18. Ibid.

19. Ibid.

20. P. Buckhart, "The effect of the alkali load of mineral water on bone metabolism: Interventional studies," *J Nutr,* vol. 138, 2008, p. 435s–37s; T. Buclin, M. Cosma, M. Appenzeller et al., "Diet acids and alkali influence calcium retention in bone," *Osteoporos Int,* vol. 12, 2001, 493–99.

21. E. Wynn, M.A. Krieg, J.M. Aeschlimann, p. Burckhardt, "Alkaline mineral water lowers bone resorption even in calcium sufficiency: Alkaline mineral water and bone metabolism," *Bone,* vol. 44, 2009, p. 120–24; E. Wynn, M.A. Krieg, S.A. Lanham-New et al., "Postgraduate Symposium: Positive influence of nutritional alkalinity on bone health," *Proc Nutr Soc,* vol. 69, 2010, 166–73.

22. Ibid.

23. C. Kousmine, *Sauvez votre corps,* Paris, Éditions J'ai lu, 1987, 629 p.

24. L.A. Frassetto, R.C. Morris Jr, D.E. Sellmeyer et al., "Diet, evolution and aging," *Eur J Nutr,* vol. 40, 2001, p. 200–13.

25. E. Wynn, M.A. Krieg, J.M. Aeschlimann and P. Burckhardt, "Alkaline mineral water lowers bone resorption even in calcium sufficiency: Alkaline mineral water and bone metabolism," *Bone,* vol. 44, 2009, p. 120–24; E. Wynn, M.A. Krieg, S.A. Lanham-New et al., "Postgraduate Symposium: Positive influence of nutritional alkalinity on bone health," *Proc Nutr Soc,* vol. 69, 2010, 166–73.

26. R. Penner, R.N. Fedorak and K.L. Madsen, "Probiotics and nutraceuticals: Non-medicinal treatments of gastrointestinal diseases," *Curr Opin Pharmacol,* vol. 5, 2005, p. 596–603; H. Tlaskalová-Hogenová, R. Stepánková, T. Hudcovic et al., "Commensal bacteria (normal microflora), mucosal immunity and chronic inflammatory and autoimmune diseases," *Immunol Lett,* vol. 93, 2004, p. 97–108.

27. B.D. Huff, "Caveat emptor: Probiotics might not be what they seem," *Fam Physician,* vol. 50, 2004, p. 583–87.

28. L.C. Allgeyer, M.J. Miller and S.Y. Lee, "Sensory and microbiological quality of yogurt drinks with prebiotics and probiotics," *J Dairy Sci,* vol. 93, 2010, p. 4471–79.

29. M. Beausoleil, N. Fortier, S. Guenette et al., "Effect of a fermented milk combining *Lactobacillus acidophilus* CL1285 and *Lactobacillus casei* in the prevention of antibiotic-associated diarrhea: A randomized, double-blind, placebo-controlled trial," *Can J Gastroenterol,* vol. 21, 2007, p. 732–36; X.W. Gao, M. Mubasher, C.Y. Fang et al., "Dose response efficacy of a proprietary probiotic formula of *Lactobacillus acidophilus* CL1285 and *Lactobacillus casei* LBC80R for antibiotic-associated diarrhea and *Clostridium difficile*-associated diarrhea prophylaxis in adult patients," *Am J Gastroenterol,* vol. 105, 2010, p. 1636–41.

30. X.W. Gao, M. Mubasher, C.Y. Fang et al., "Dose-response efficacy of a proprietary probiotic formula of *Lactobacillus acidophilus* CL1285 and *Lactobacillus casei* LBC80R for antibiotic-associated diarrhea and *Clostridium difficile*-associated diarrhea prophylaxis in adult patients," *Am J Gastroenterol,* vol. 105, 2010, p. 1636–41.

31. D. Thomas, "The mineral depletion of foods available to us as a nation (1940–2002): A review of the 6th edition of McCance and Widdowson," *Nutr Health,* vol. 19, 2007, p. 21–55.

32. A.N. Mayer, "Historical change in the mineral content of fruits and vegetables," *British Food Journal,* vol. 99, 1997, p. 207–11.

33. Ibid.

34. D. Thomas, "The mineral depletion of foods available to us as a nation (1940–2002): A review of the 6th edition of McCance and Widdowson," *Nutr Health,* vol. 19, 2007, p. 21–55.

35. Ibid.

36. Ibid.

37. S. Bengmark, "Ecological control of the gastrointestinal tract: The role of probiotic flora," *Gut,* vol. 42, 1998, p. 2–7.

38. D.R. Jacobs, Jr., M.D. Gross and L.C. Tapsell, "Food synergy: An operational concept for understanding nutrition," *Am J Clin Nutr,* vol. 89 (suppl.), 2009, p. 1543s–48s.

39. Ibid.

40. R.H. Liu, J. Liu and B. Chen, "Apples prevent mammary tumors in rats," *J Agric Food Chem,* vol. 53, 2005, p. 2341–43.

41. M. Stacewicz-Sapuntzakis and P.E. Bowen, "Role of lycopene and tomato products in prostate health," *Biochim Biophys Acta,* vol. 1740, 2005, p. 202–05; T.W. Boileau, Z. Lia, S. Kim et al., "Prostate carcinogenesis in n-methyl–n-nitrosourea (nmu)-testosterone-treated rats fed tomato powder, lycopene, or energy-restricted diets," *J Nail Cancer Inst,* vol. 95, 2003, p. 1578–86.

42. F. Van Wijk, S. Nierkens, I. Hassing et al., "The effect of the food matrix on in vivo immune responses to purified peanut allergens," *Toxicol Sci,* vol. 86, 2005, p. 333–41.

43. niii state-of-the-science panel, "National Institutes of Health state-of-the-science conference statement: Multivitamin/mineral supplements and chronic disease prevention," *Annals of Internal Medicine,* vol. 145, 2006, p. 364–70; E.R. Miller, R. Pastor-Barriuso, D. Dalai et al., "Meta-analysis: High-dosage vitamin E supplementation may increase all-cause mortality," *Ann Intern Med,* vol. 142, 2005, p. 37–46.

44. nih state-of-the-science panel, "National Institutes of Health state-of-the-science conference statement: Multivitamin/mineral supplements and chronic disease prevention," *Annals of Internal Medicine,* vol. 145, 2006, p. 364–70.

45. K. Barnard and C. Colon-Emeric, "Extraskeletal effects of vitamin D in older adults: Cardiovascular disease, mortality, mood, and cognition," *Am J Geriatr Pharmacother,* vol. 8, 2010, p. 4–33.

46. B. Dawson-Hugues, S.S. Harris, E.A. Krall et al., "Effect of calcium and vitamin D supplementation on bone density in men and women 65 years of age or older," *N Engl J Med,* vol. 337, 1997, p. 670–76.

47. M.C. Chapuy, M.E. Arlot, F. Duboeuf et al., "Vitamin D3 and calcium to prevent hip fractures in the elderly women," *N Engl J Med,* vol. 327, 1992, p. 1637–42.

48. G. Bergman, T. Fan, J.T. McFertridge et al., "Efficacy of vitamin D3 supplementation in preventing fractures in elderly women: A meta-analysis," *Curr Med Res Opin,* vol. 26, 2010, p. 1193–1201.

49. G. Buhr and C.W. Bales, "Nutritional supplements for older adults: Review and recommendations: Part I," *J Nutr Elder,* vol. 28, 2009, p. 5–29.

50. M.F. Holick, "The vitamin D deficiency pandemic and consequences for nonskeletal health: Mechanisms of action," *Molecular Aspects of Medicine,* vol. 29, 2008, p. 361–68.

51. M. Peterlik and H.S. Cross, "Vitamin D and calcium insufficiency-related chronic diseases: Molecular and cellular pathophysiology," *Eur J Clin Nutr,* vol. 63, 2009, p. 1377–86.

52. L.A. Merlino, J. Curtis, T.R. Mikuls et al., "Vitamin D intake is inversely associated with rheumatoid arthritis: Results from the Iowa Women's Health Study," *Arthritis Rheum,* 50, 2004, p. 72–77.

53. T.E. McAlindon, D.T. Felson, Y. Zhang et al., "Relation of dietary intake and serum levels of vitamin D to progression of osteoarthritis of the knee among participants in the Framingham Study," *Ann Intern Med,* 125, 1996, p. 353–59.

54. G. Sigurdsson, L. Franzson, L. Steingrimsdottir et al., "The association between parathyroid hormone, vitamin D and bone mineral density in 70-year-old icelandic women," *Osteoporos Int,* vol. 11, 2000, p. 1031–35.

55. R.P. Heaney, "Is the paradigm shifting?" *Bone,* vol. 33, 2003, p. 457–65.

56. L. Steingrimsdottir, O. Gunnarsson, O.S. Indridason et al., "Relationship between serum parathyroid hormone levels, vitamin D sufficiency, and calcium intake," *JAMA,* vol. 294, 2005, p. 2336–41.

57. G. Buhr and C.W. Bales, "Nutritional supplements for older adults: Review and recommendations: Part I," *J Nutr Elder,* vol. 28, 2009, p. 5–29.

58. Ibid.

59. J. Martel-Pettetier, S. Kwan Tat and J.-P. Pelletier, "Effects of chondroitin sulfate in the pathophysiology of the osteoarthritic joint: A narrative review," *Osteoarthritis Cartilage,* vol. 18 (suppl.1), 2010, p. s7–s11.

60. Ibid.

61. J. Monfort, J. Martel-Pelletier, J.-P. Pelletier, "Chondroitin sulfate for symptomatic osteoarthritis: Critical appraisal of meta-analyses," *Curr Med Res Opin,* vol. 24, 2008, p. 1303–08.

62. Y.H. Lee, J.H. Woo, S.J. Choi et al., "Effect of glucosamine or chondroitin sulfate on the osteoarthritis progression: A meta-analysis," *Rheumatol Int,* vol. 30, 2010, p. 357–63.

63. J. Martel-Pettetier, S. Kwan Tat and J.-P. Pelletier, "Effects of chondroitin sulfate in the pathophysiology of the osteoarthritic joint: A narrative review," *Osteoarthritis Cartilage,* vol. 18 (suppl.1), 2010, p. s7–s11.

64. J.Y. Reginster, "The efficacy of glucosamine sulfate in osteoarthritis: Financial and nonfinancial conflict of interest," *Arthritis Rheum,* vol. 56, 2007, p. 2105–10.

65. J.B. Houpt, R. McMilan, C. Wein et al., "Effect of glucosamine hydrochloride in the treatment of pain of osteoarthritis of the knee," *J Rheumatol,* vol. 26, 1999, p. 2423–30; D.O. Clegg, D.J. Reda, C.L. Harris et al., "Glucosamine, chondroitin sulfate, and the two in combination for painful knee osteoarthritis," *N Engl J Med,* vol. 354, 2006, p. 795–808.

66. G. Herrero-Beaumont, J.A. Roman Ivorra, M. Del Carmen Trabado et al., "Glucosamine sulfate in the treatment of knee osteoarthritis symptoms: A randomized, double-blind, placebo-controlled study using acetaminophen as a side comparator," *Arthritis Rheum,* vol. 56, 2007, p. 555–67.

67. J.Y. Reginster, "The efficacy of glucosamine sulfate in osteoarthritis: Financial and nonfinancial conflict of interest," *Arthritis Rheum,* vol. 56, 2007, p. 2105–10.

68. C.Y. Chang, D.S. Ke and J.Y. Chen, "Essential fatty acids and human brain," *Acta Neurol Taiwan,* vol. 18, 2009, p. 231–41.

69. The National Diet-Heart Study Final Report, *Circulation,* vol. 37, 1968, p. 11–428.

70. F.A. Kummerow, "The negative effects of hydrogenated trans fat and what to do about them," *Artherosclerosis,* vol. 205, 2009, p. 458–65.

71. Ibid.

72. L. Ricciuto, K. Lin and V. Tarasuk, "A comparison of the fat composition and prices of margarines between 2002 and 2006, when new Canadian labelling regulations came into effect," *Public Health Nutrition,* vol. 12, 2008, p. 1270–75.

73. M.J. Albers, L.J. Harnack, L.M. Stephen et al., "2006 marketplace survey of trans-fatty acid content of margarines and butters, cookies and snack cakes, and savory snacks," *J Am Diet Assoc,* vol. 108, 2008, p. 367–70.

74. Ibid.

75. S. Innis, T. Green and T. Halsey, "Variability in the trans fatty acid content of foods within a food category: Implications for estimation of dietary trans fatty acid intakes," *J Am Coll Nutr,* vol. 18, 1999, p. 255–260.(OK)

76. C.M. Skeaff, "Feasibility of recommending certain replacement or alternative fats," *Eur J Clin Nutr,* vol. 63, 2009, p. s34–s49.

77. S.I. Elias and S.M. Innis, "Bakery foods are the major dietary source of trans-fatty acids among pregnant women with diets providing 30 percent energy from fat," *J Am Diet Assoc,* vol. 102, 2002, p. 46–51.

78. A.H. Zevenbergen, A. de Bree, M. Zeelenberg et al., "Foods with a high fat quality are essential for healthy diets," *Ann Nutr Metab,* vol. 54, 2009, p. 15–24.

79. Ibid.

80. M. Collino, "High dietary fructose intake: Sweet or bitter life?" *World J Diabetes,* vol. 2, 2011, p. 77–81.

81. R.J. Johnson, L.G. Sanchez-Lozada and T. Nakagawa, "The effect of fructose on renal biology and disease," www.ncbi.nlm.nih.gov/pubmed/21115612, *J Am Soc Nephrol,* vol. 21, 2010, p. 2036–2039.

82. A. Brymora, M. Flisinski, R.J. Johnson et al., "Low-fructose diet lowers blood pressure and inflammation in patients with chronic kidney disease," *Nephrol Dial Transplant,* vol. 27, 2012, p. 608–12.

83. Ibid., note 26.

84. Ibid., note 25.

85. G. Suarez, R. Rajaram, A.L. Oronsky and M.A. Gawinowicz, "Nonenzymatic glycation of bovine serum albumin by fructose (fructation): Comparison with the Maillard reaction initiated by glucose," *J Biol Chem,* vol. 264, 1989, p. 3674–79.

86. M. Kretowicz, R.J. Johnson, T. Ishimoto et al., "The impact of fructose on renal function and blood pressure," *Int J Nephrol,* 2011:315879. Epub July 17, 2011.

87. M. Madero, J.C. Arriaga, D. Jalal et al., "The effect of two energy restricted diets, a low-fructose diet versus a moderate natural fructose diet, on weight loss and metabolic syndrome parameters: A randomized controlled trial," *Metabolism,* vol. 60, no. 11, 2011, p. 1551–9.

88. D.I. Jalal, G. Smits, R.J. Johnson and M. Chonchol, "Increased fructose associates with elevated blood pressure," *J Am Soc Nephrol,* vol. 21, 2010, p. 1543–49. Epub July 1, 2010.

89. Ibid., note 27.

90. Ibid., note 33.

91. D. Stellato, L.F. Morrone, C. Di Giorgio and L. Gesualdo , "Uric acid: A starring role in the intricate scenario of metabolic syndrome with cardio-renal damage?" *Intern Emerg Med,* vol. 7, 2012, p. 5–8.

92. Ibid., note 31.

93. Ibid., note 26.

7 THE IMMUNE SYSTEM'S STRATEGIES IN CHRONIC INFLAMMATORY DISEASES

1. J. Seignalet, *L'Alimentation ou la troisième médecine,* 5e éd., Paris, Office d'Edition Impression Librairie, 2004, 660 p.

2. W.E. Paul et al., *Fundamental Immunology,* 6th ed., New York, Raven Press, 2007, 1632 p.

3. C.A. Janeway, K. Murphy, P. Travers et al., *Immunobiologie,* 3e éd., Paris, De Boech, 2009, 922 p.

4. B. Sears, *Le régime anti-inflammatoire. Comment vaincre ce mal silencieux qui détruit votre santé,* Montréal, Les Éditions de l'Homme, 2006, 411 p.

5. Ibid.

6. Ibid.

7. Ibid.
8. M.P. Lehucher-Michel, J.F. Lesgards, O. Delubac et al., "Oxidative stress and human disease: Current knowledge and perspectives for prevention," *Presse Med,* vol. 30, 2001, p. 1076–81.
9. G. Lettre and J.D. Rioux, "Autoimmune diseases: Insights from genome-wide association studies," *Hum Mol Genet,* vol. 17, 2008, p. R116–21.
10. T. Shiina, H. Inoko and J.K. Kulski, "An update of the HLA genomic region, locus information and disease associations: 2004," *Tissue Antigens,* vol. 64, 2004, p. 631–49.

8   RHEUMATOID ARTHRITIS AND THE HYPOTOXIC DIET

1. S.M. Dai, X.H. Han, D.B. Zha et al., "Prevalence of rheumatic symptoms, rheumatoid arthritis, ankylosing spondylitis, and gout in Shanghai, China: A COPCORD study," *J Rheumatol,* vol. 30, 2003, p. 2090–91; O.O. Adelowo, O. Ojo, I. Oduenyi et al., "Rheumatoid arthritis among Nigerians: The first 200 patients from a rheumatology clinic," *Clin Rheumatol,* vol. 29, 2010, p. 593–97.
2. C. Ramos-Remus, G. Sierra-Jimenez, K. Skeith et al., "Latitude gradient influences the age of onset in rheumatoid arthritis patients ," *Clin Rheumatol,* vol. 26, 2007, p. 1725–28.
3. P.K. Gregersen, J. Silver and R.J. Winchester, "The shared epitope hypothesis: An approach to understanding the molecular genetics of susceptibility to rheumatoid arthritis," *Arthritis Rheum,* vol. 30, 1987, p. 1205–13; L. Klareskog, U. Forsum, A. Scheynius et al., "Evidence in support of a self-perpetuating HLADR-dependent delayed-type cell reaction in rheumatoid arthritis," *Proc Natl Acad Sci USA,* vol. 79, 1982, p. 3632–36.
4. C. Vignal, A.T. Bansal, D.J. Balding et al., "Genetic association of the major histocompatibility complex with rheumatoid arthritis implicates two non-DRB1 loci," *Arthritis Rheum,* vol. 60, 2009, p. 2207.
5. M. Bukhari, M. Lunt, B.J. Harrison et al., "Rheumatoid factor is the major predictor of increasing severity of radiographic erosions in rheumatoid arthritis: Results from the Norfolk Arthritis Register Study, a large inception cohort," *Arthritis Rheum,* vol. 46, 2002, p. 906–12.
6. P.F. Whiting, N. Smidt, J.A. Sterne et al., "Systematic review: Accuracy of anti-citrullinated peptide antibodies for diagnosing rheumatoid arthritis," *Ann Intern Med,* vol. 152, 2010, p. 456–64.
7. G.J. Pruijn, A. Wilk and W.J. van Venrooij, "The use of citrullinated peptides and proteins for the diagnosis of rheumatoid arthritis," *Arthritis Res Ther,* vol. 12, 2010, p. 203; N. Vuilleumier, S. Bas, S. Pagano et al., "Anti-apolipoprotein A-1 IgG predict major cardiovascular events in patients with rheumatoid arthritis," *Arthritis Rheum,* vol. 62, 2010, p. 2640–50.

8. C. Turesson, W.M. O'Fallon, C.S. Crowson et al., "Extra-articular disease manifestations in rheumatoid arthritis: Incidence trends and risk factors over 46 years," *Ann Rheum Dis,* vol. 62, 2003, p. 722–27; J.M. Berthelot, H.J. Bernelot-Moens, M. Klarlund et al., "Differences in understanding and application of 1987 ACR criteria for rheumatoid arthritis and 1991 ESSG criteria for spondylarthropathy: A pilot survey," *Clin Exp Rheumatol,* vol. 20, 2002, p. 145–50.

9. M.A. van Boekel, E.R. Vossenaar, F.H. van den Hoogen et al., "Autoantibody systems in rheumatoid arthritis: Specificity, sensitivity and diagnostic value," *Arthritis Res,* vol. 4, 2002, p. 87–93; S. Bas, S. Ganevay, O. Meyer et al.,"Anti-cyclic citrullinated peptide antibodies, IgM and IgA rheumatoid factors in the diagnosis and prognosis of rheumatoid arthritis," *Rheumatology* (Oxford), vol. 42, 2003, p. 677–80.

10. T.K. Kvien, "Epidemiology and burden of illness of rheumatoid arthritis," *Pharmacoeconomics,* vol. 22 (2 Suppl. 1), 2004, p. 1–12; N. Graudal, "The natural history and prognosis of rheumatoid arthritis: Association of radiographic outcome with process variables, joint motion and immune proteins," *Scand J Rheumatol,* vol. 118 (Suppl.), 2004, p. 1–38.

11. A.G. Pratt, J.D. Isaacs and D.L. Mattey, "Current concepts in the pathogenesis of early rheumatoid arthritis," *Best Pract Res Clin Rheumatol,* vol. 23, 2009, p. 37–48.

12. I. Hafström, B. Ringertz, A. Spångberg et al., "A vegan diet free of gluten improves the signs and symptoms of rheumatoid arthritis: The effects on arthritis correlate with a reduction in antibodies to food antigens," *Rheumatology* (Oxford), vol. 40, 2001, p. 1175–79; A.C. Elkan, B. Sjöberg, B. Kolsrud et al., "Gluten-free vegan diet induces decreased LDL and oxidized LDL levels and raised atheroprotective natural antibodies against phosphorylcholine in patients with rheumatoid arthritis: A randomized study," *Arthritis Res Ther,* vol. 10, 2008, p. R34. Available for free: arthritis-research.com/content/10/2/R34 (8 p.).

13. A.G. Pratt, J.D. Isaacs and D.L.Mattey, "Current concepts in the pathogenesis of early rheumatoid arthritis," *Best Pract Res Clin Rheumatol,* vol. 23, 2009, p. 37–48.

14. A.H. van der Helm-van Mil, T.W.J. Huizinga, G.M. Schreuder et al., "An independent role of protective HLA class I alleles in rheumatoid arthritis severity and susceptibility," *Arthritis Rheum,*vol. 52, 2005, p. 2637–44.

15. J.E. Oliver and A.J. Silman, "Risk factors for the development of rheumatoid arthritis" *Scand J Rheumatol,* vol. 35, 2006, p. 169–74.

16. E.W. Karlson, L.A. Mandl, S.E. Hankinson et al., "Do breast-feeding and other reproductive factors influence future risk of rheumatoid arthritis? Results from the Nurses' Health Study," *Arthritis Rheum,* vol. 50, 2004, p. 3458–67.

17. M. Cutolo and S. Accardo, "Sex hormones, HLA and rheumatoid arthritis," *Clin Exp Rheumatol,* vol. 9, 1991, p. 641–46; M. Schmidt, H. Naurmann, C. Weidler et al., "Inflammation and sex hormone metabolism," *Ann NY Acad Sci,* vol. 1069, 2006, p. 236–46.

18. D. Hutchinson, L. Shepstone, R. Moots et al., "Heavy cigarette smoking is strongly associated with rheumatoid arthritis (RA), particularly in patients without a family history of RA," *Ann Rheum Dis,* vol. 60, 2001, p. 223–27.

19. A.J. Silman, J. Newman and A.J. Macgregor, "Cigarette smoking increases the risk of rheumatoid arthritis: Results from a nationwide study of disease-discordant twins," *Arthritis Rheum,* vol. 39, 1996, p. 732–35.

20. N.G. Papadopoulos, Y. Alamanos, P.V. Voulgari et al., "Does cigarette smoking influence disease expression, activity and severity in early rheumatoid arthritis patients?" *Clin Exp Rheumatol,* vol. 23, 2005, p. 861–66.

21. S.M. Carty, N. Snowden, A.J.Silman, "Should infection still be considered as the most likely triggering factor for rheumatoid arthritis ?" *J Rheumatol,* vol. 30, 2003, p. 425–29.

22. H. Tiwana, C. Wilson, P. Cunningham et al., "Antibodies to four gram-negative bacteria in rheumatoid arthritis which share sequences with the rheumatoid arthritis susceptibility motif," *Br J Rheumatol,* vol. 35, 1996, p. 592–94.

23. N. Balandraud, J. Roudier and C. Roudier, "Esptein-Barr virus and rheumatoid arthritis," *Autoimmun Rev,* vol. 3, 2004, p. 362–67.

24. T. Rashid and A. Ebringer, "Rheumatoid arthritis is linked to *Proteus:* The evidence," *Clin Rheumatol,* vol. 26, 2007, p. 1036–43.

25. C. Wilson, T. Rashid, H. Tiwana et al., "Cytotoxicity responses to peptide antigens in rheumatoid arthritis and ankylosing spondylitis," *J Rheumatol,* vol. 30, 2003, p. 972–78; A. Ebringer, T. Rashid and C. Wilson, "Rheumatoid arthritis, Proteus, anti-CCP antibodies and Karl Popper," *Autoimmun Rev,* vol. 9, 2010, p. 216–223

26. C.J. Henderson and R.S. Panush,"Diets, dietary supplements, and nutritional therapies in rheumatic diseases," *Rheum Dis Clin North Am,* vol. 25, 1999, p. 937–68.

27. Ibid.

28. D.J. Pattison, R.A. Harrison and D.P. Symmons, "The role of diet in susceptibility to rheumatoid arthritis: A systematic review," *J Rheumatol,* vol. 31, 2004, p. 1310–19.

29. P.C. Calder and P. Yaqoob, "Understanding omega-3 polyunsaturated fatty acids," *Postgrad Med,* vol. 121, 2009, p. 148–57.

30. D.J. Pattison, R.A. Harrison and D.P. Symmons, "The role of diet in susceptibility to rheumatoid arthritis: A systematic review," *J Rheumatol,* vol. 31, 2004, p. 1310–19.

31. L.G. Darlington, N.W. Ramsey and J.R. Mansfield, "Placebo-controlled, blind study of dietary manipulation therapy in rheumatoid arthritis," *Lancet,* vol. 1, 1986, p. 236–38.

32. L.G. Darlington, N.W. Ramsey and J.R. Mansfield, "Placebo-controlled, blind study of dietary manipulation therapy in rheumatoid arthritis," *Lancet,* vol. 1, 1986, p. 236–38; L.G. Darlington and N.W. Ramsey, "Review of dietary therapy for rheumatoid arthritis ," *Br J Rheumatol,* vol. 32, 1993, p. 507–14.

33. G.E. Hein, M. Köhler, P. Œznep et al., "The advanced glycation end product pentosidine correlates to IL-6 and other relevant inflammatory markers in rheumatoid arthritis," *Rheumatol Int,* vol. 26, 2005, p. 137–41; T. Miyata, W. Ishiguro, Y. Yasuda et al., "Increased pentosidine, an advanced glycation end product, in plasma and synovial fluid from patients with rheumatoid arthritis and its relation with inflammatory markers," *Biochem Biophys Res Commun,* vol. 244, 1998, p. 45–49.

34. L. Sköldstam, L. Hagfors and G. Johansson, "An experimental study of a Mediterranean diet intervention for patients with rheumatoid arthritis," *Ann Rheum Dis,* vol. 62, 2003, p. 208–14; G. McKellar, E. Morrison, A. McEntegart et al., "A pilot study of a Mediterranean type diet intervention in female patients with rheumatoid arthritis living in areas of social deprivation in Glasgow," *Ann Rheum Dis,* vol. 66, 2007, p. 1239–43.

35. L. Sköldstam, L. Hagfors and G.Johansson, "An experimental study of a Mediterranean diet intervention for patients with rheumatoid arthritis," *Ann Rheum Dis,* vol. 62, 2003, p. 208–14.

36. M. De Lorgeril, S. Renaud, N. Mamelle et al., "Mediterranean alphalinolenic acid rich diet in secondary prevention of coronary heart disease," *Lancet,* vol. 343, 1994, p. 1454–59.

37. L. Hagfors, I. Nilsson, L. Sköldstam et al., "Fat intake and composition of fatty acids in serum phospholipids in a randomized, controlled, Mediterranean dietary intervention study on patients with rheumatoid arthritis," *Nurt Metab* (Lond), vol. 10, 2005, p. 2–26.

38. G. McKellar, E. Morrison, A. McEntegart et al.,"A pilot study of a Mediterranean-type diet intervention in female patients with rheumatoid arthritis living in areas of social deprivation in Glasgow," *Ann Rheum Dis,* vol. 66, 2007, p. 1239–43.

39. T.C. Campbell and T.M. Campbell, *Le Rapport Campbell. Révélations stupéfiantes sur les liens entre L'Alimentation et la santé à long terme,* Outremont, Éditions Ariane, 2008, 488 p.; C.T. Campbell and T.M. Campbell. *The China Study.* Benbella Books, Dallas, 2006.

40. Ibid.

9 OTHER AUTOIMMUNE DISEASES THAT RESPONDED POSITIVELY TO THE HYPOTOXIC DIET

1. www.arthritis.ca; V.K. Dik, M.J.L. Peters, M.A.C. Dijkmans et al., "The relationship between disease-related characteristics and conduction disturbances in ankylosing spondylitis," *Scand J Rheumatol,* vol. 39, 2010, p. 38–41.

2. M.A. Brown, S.H. Laval, S. Brophy et al., "Recurrence risk modelling of the genetic susceptibility to ankylosing spondylitis," *Ann Rheum Dis,* vol. 59, 2000, p. 883–86.

3. M.H. Sombekke, D. Arteta, M.A. van de Wiel et al., "Analysis of multiple candidate genes in association with phenotypes of multiple sclerosis," *Mult Scler,* vol. 16, 2010, p. 652–59.

4. R.A. Marrie, N. Yu, J. Blanchard et al., "The rising prevalence and changing age distribution of multiple sclerosis in Manitoba," *Neurology,* vol. 74, 2010, p. 465–71.

5. A. Ebringer, T. Rashid and C. Wilson, "Bovine spongiform encephalopathy, multiple sclerosis, and creutzfeldt-jakob disease are probably autoimmune diseases evoked by Acinetobacter bacteria," *Ann NY Acad Sci,* vol. 1050, 2005, p. 417–28.

10 SEIGNALET'S THEORY ON THE PHENOMENON OF TISSUE DEPOSITION AS THE CAUSE OF CERTAIN CHRONIC INFLAMMATORY DISEASES

1. A.D. Woolf and B. Pfleger, "Burden of major musculoskeletal conditions," *Bull World Health Organ,* vol. 81, 2003, p. 646–56.

2. R.C. Lawrence, C.G. Helmick, F.C. Arnett et al., "Estimates of the prevalence of arthritis and selected musculoskeletal disorders in the United States," *Arthritis Rheum,* vol. 41, 1998, p. 778–99.

3. M.B. Goldring and S.R. Goldring, "Osteoarthritis," *J Cell Physiol,* vol. 213, 2007, p. 626–34.

4. P. Qvist, A.C. Bay-Jensen, C. Christiansen et al., "The disease modifying osteoarthritis drug (DMOAD): Is it in the horizon ?" *Pharmacol Res,* vol. 58, 2008, p. 1–7.

5. B. Haraoui, J.-P. Pelletier, J.-M. Cloutier et al., "Synovial membrane histology and immunopathology in rheumatoid arthritis and osteoarthritis: In vivo effects of antirheumatic drugs," *Arthritis Rheum,* vol. 34, 1991, p. 153–63; R.R. Da, Y. Qin, D. Baeten et al., "B cell clonal expansion and somatic hypermutation of Ig variable heavy chain genes in the synovial membrane of patients with osteoarthritis," *J Immunol,* vol. 178, 2007, p. 557–65.

6. S. Ashraf and D.A. Walsh, "Angiogenesis in osteoarthritis," *Curr Opin Rheumatol,* vol. 20, 2008, p. 573–80; J. Martel-Pelletier and J.-P. Pelletier, "Is osteoarthritis a disease involving only cartilage or other articular tissues?" *Joint Diseases and Related Surgery,* vol. 21, 2010, p. 2–14.

7. S. Ashraf and D.A. Walsh, "Angiogenesis in osteoarthritis," *Curr Opin Rheumatol,* vol. 20, 2008, p. 573–80.

8. D.A. Walsh, C.S. Bonnet, E.L. Turner et al., "Angiogenesis in the synovium and at the osteochondral junction in osteoarthritis," *Osteoarthritis Cartilage,* vol. 15, 2007, p. 743–51.

9. S. Ashraf and D.A. Walsh, "Angiogenesis in osteoarthritis," *Curr Opin Rheumatol,* vol. 20, 2008, p. 573–80.

10. S. Ashraf and D.A. Walsh, "Angiogenesis in osteoarthritis," *Curr Opin Rheumatol,* vol. 20, 2008, p. 573–80; D.A. Walsh, C.S. Bonnet, E.L. Turner et al., "Angiogenesis in the synovium and at the osteochondral junction in osteoarthritis," *Osteoarthritis Cartilage,* vol. 15, 2007, p. 743–51.

11. R.D. Leslie, H. Beyan, P. Sawtell et al., "Level of an advanced glycated end products is genetically determined: A study of normal twins," *Diabetes,* vol. 52, 2003, p. 2441–44.

12. N. Verzijl, J. DeGroot, S.R. Thorpe et al., "Effect of collagen turnover on the accumulation of advanced glycation end products," *J Bio Chem,* vol. 275, 2000, p. 39027–31.

13. V. Prakash Reddy and A. Beyaz, "Inhibitors of the Maillard reaction and AGE breakers as therapeutics for multiple diseases," *Drug Discov Today,* vol. 11, 2006, p. 646–54.

14. J. DeGroot, "The AGE of the matrix: Chemistry, consequence and cure," *Curr Opin Pharmacol,* vol. 4, 2004, p. 301–05.

15. H. Vlassara, "Advanced glycation in health and disease: Role of the modern environment," *Ann NY Acad Sci,* vol. 1043, 2005, p. 452–60.

16. J. DeGroot, "The AGE of the matrix: Chemistry, consequence and cure," *Curr Opin Pharmacol,* vol. 4, 2004, p. 301–05; J. DeGroot, N. Verzijl, M.J. Wenting-van Wijk et al., "Accumulation of advanced glycation end products as a molecular mechanism for aging as a risk factor in osteoarthritis," *Arthritis Rheum,* vol. 50, 2004, p. 1207–15.

17. F. Wolfe, "The relation between tender points and fibromyalgia symptom variables: Evidence that fibromyalgia is not a discrete disorder in the clinic," *Ann Rheum Dis,* vol. 56, 1997, p. 268–71.

18. R.M. Bennett, J. Jones, D.C. Turk et al., "An internet survey of 2,596 people with fibromyalgia," *BMC Musculoskelet Disord,* vol. 8, 2007, p. 27. Available for free: www.biomedcentral.com/1471-2474/8/27.

19. D.J. Clauw, "Fibromyalgia: An Overview," *Am J Med,* vol. 122, 2009, p. 1–16.

20. Ibid.

21. D. J. Clauw, "Fibromyalgia: An Overview," *Am J Med,* vol. 122, 2009, p. 1–16; V. De Silva, A. El-Metwally, E. Ernst et al., "Evidence for the efficacy of complementary and alternative medicines in the management of

fibromyalgia: A systematic review," *Rheumatology* (Oxford), vol. 49, 2010, p. 1063–68.

22. V.S. Malik, B.M. Popkin, G.A. Bray et al., "Sugar-sweetened beverages, obesity, type 2 diabetes mellitus, and cardiovascular disease risk," *Circulation,* vol. 121, 2010, p. 1356–64.

23. S.M. Ruchat, M.C. Vohl, S.J. Weisnagel et al., "Combining genetic markers and clinical risk factors improves the risk assessment of impaired glucose metabolism," *Ann Med,* vol. 42, 2010, p. 196–206.

24. S.J. Kenny, R.E. Aubert and L.S. Geiss, "Prevalence and incidence of non-insulin-dependent diabetes," in National Diabetes Data Group (dir.), *Diabetes in America,* 2nd ed., Washington, DC, National Institute of Diabetes and Digestive and Kidney Disease, 1995.

25. C.L. Leibson, P.C. O'Brien, E. Atkinson et al., "Relative contributions of incidence and survival to increasing prevalence of adult-onset diabetes mellitus: A population-based study," *Am J Epidemiol,* vol. 146, 1997, p. 12–21.

26. J.P. Bastard, M. Maachi, C. Lagathu et al., "Recent advances in the relationship between obesity, inflammation, and insulin resistance," *Eur Cytokine Netw,* vol. 17, 2006, p. 4–12.

27. L. Duvnjak and M. Duvnjak, "The metabolic syndrome: An ongoing story," *J Physio Pharmacol,* vol. 60, 2009, p. 19–24.

28. Ibid.

29. W.T. Cefalu, "The physiologic role of incretin hormones: Clinical applications," *J Am Osteopath ss,* vol. 110, 2010, p. S8–S14.

11   DISEASES OF ELIMINATION

1. N. Rajendran and D. Kumar, "Role of diet in the management of inflammatory bowel disease," *World J Gastroenterol,* vol. 16, 2010, p. 1442–48.

2. V. Binder, "Epidemiology of IBD during the twentieth century: An integrated view," *Best Pract Res Clin Gastroenterol,* vol. 18, 2004, p. 463–79.

3. P. Laszlo Lakatos, "Recent trends in the epidemiology of inflammatory bowel diseases: Up or down?" *World Gastroenterol,* vol. 14, 2006, p. 6102–08; X. Han, "Intestinal permeability as a clinical surrogate endpoint in the development of future Crohn's disease therapies," *Recent Pat Inflamm Allergy Drug Discov,* vol. 4, 2010, p. 159–76.

4. G.M. White, "Recent findings in the epidemiologic evidence, classification, and subtypes of acne vulgaris," *J Am Acad Dermatol,* vol. 39, 1998, p. S34–S37.

5. H.R. Ferdowsian, S. Levin, "Does diet really affect acne?" *Skin Therapy lett,* vol. 15, 2010, p. 1–2.

6. Ibid.

7. Ibid.

8. Food and Drug Administration, HHS, "Classification of benzoyl peroxide as safe and effective and revision of labeling to drug facts format; topical acne drug products for over-the-counter human use; final rule," *Fed Regist,* vol. 75, 2010, p. 9767–77; A.D. Katsambas and C. Dessinioti, "Hormonal therapy for acne: Why not as first line therapy? Facts and controversies," *Clin Dermatol,* vol. 28, 2010, p. 17–23; G.F. Webster, "Light and laser therapy for acne: Sham or science? Facts and controversies," *Clinics in Dermatology,* vol. 28, 2010, p. 31–33.

9. J.M. Spergel, "Epidemiology of atopic dermatitis and atopic march in children," *Immunol Allergy Clin North Am,* vol. 30, 2010, p. 269–80.

10. S.J. Brown and W.H. McLean, "Eczema genetics: Current state of knowledge and future goals," *J Invest Dermatol,* vol. 129, 2009, p. 543–52.

11. M. Wang, C. Karlsson, C. Olsson et al., "Reduced diversity in the early fecal microbiota of infants with atopic eczema," *J Allergy Clin Immunol,* vol. 121, 2008, p. 129–34.

12. S.G. Plotz and J. Ring, "What's new in atopic eczema?" *Expert Opin Emerg Drugs,* vol. 15, 2010, p. 249–67.

13. D.H. Broide, "Molecular and cellular mechanisms of allergic disease," *J Allergy Clin Immunol,* vol. 108, 2001, p. S65–S71.

14. S.N. Georas, F. Rezaee, L. Lerner et al., "Dangerous allergens: Why some allergens are bad actors," *Curr Allergy Asthma Rep,* vol. 10, 2010, p. 92–98.

15. B. Bloom, R.A. Cohen and G. Freeman, "Summary health statistics for U.S. children: National Health Interview Survey, 2007," *Vital Health Stat,* vol. 10, 2009, p. 1–80.

16. T. To, S. Dell, P. Dick et al., "The burden of illness experienced by young children associated with asthma: A population-based cohort study," *J Asthma,* vol. 45, 2008, p. 45–49.

17. D.H. Broide, "Molecular and cellular mechanisms of allergic disease," *J Allergy Clin Immunol,* vol. 108, 2001, p. S65–S71.

18. D.K. Agrawal and Z. Shao, "Pathogenesis of Allergic Airway Inflammation," *Curr Allergy Asthma Rep,* vol. 10, 2010, p. 39–48.

19. Z. Liu, N. Li and J. Neu, "Tight junctions, leaky intestines, and pediatric diseases," *Acta oediatrica,* vol. 94, 2005, p. 386–93.

20. P.G. Jackson, M.H. Lessof, R.W. Baker et al., "Intestinal permeability in patients with eczema and food allergy," *Lancet,* vol. 1, 1981, p. 1285–86.

21. A. Benard, P. Desreumeaux, D. Huglo et al., "Increased intestinal permeability in bronchial asthma," *J Allergy Clin Immunol,* vol. 97, 1996, p. 1173–78.

12 DRUGS USED TO TREAT INFLAMMATORY DISEASE

1. D.F. Legler, M. Bruckner, W. Uetzvon Allmen et al., "Prostaglandin E2 at new glance: Novel insights in functional diversity offer therapeutic chances," *Int J Biochem Cell Biol,* vol. 42, 2010, p. 198–201.

2. P.C. Calder, "Polyunsaturated fatty acids and inflammatory processes: New twists in an old tale," *Biochimie,* vol. 91, 2009, p. 791–95.

3. D.F. Legler, M. Bruckner, W. Uetzvon Allmen et al., "Prostaglandin E2 at new glance: Novel insights in functional diversity offer therapeutic chances," *Int J Biochem Cell Biol,* vol. 42, 2010, p. 198–201.

4. P.C. Calder, "Polyunsaturated fatty acids and inflammatory processes: New twists in an old tale," *Biochimie,* vol. 91, 2009, p. 791–95.

5. B. Sears, *Le régime anti-inflammatoire. Comment vaincre ce mal silencieux qui détruit votre santé,* Montréal, Éditions de l'Homme, 2006, 411 p.; L. Gannari and J.P. Bilezikian, "Glucocorticoid-induced osteoporosis: Hope in the HORIZON," *Lancet,* vol. 373, 2009, p. 1225–26; N.E. Lane and W. Yao, "Glucocorticoid-induced bone fragility," *Ann NY Acad Sci,* vol. 1192, 2010, p. 81–83.

6. J. Pergolizzi, R.H. Böger, K. Budd et al., "Opioids and the managements of chronic severe pain in the elderly: Consensus statement of an International Expert Panel with focus on the six clinically most often used World Health Organization Step III opioids (buprenorphine, fentanyl, hydromorphone, methadone, morphine, oxycodone)," *Pain Pract,* vol. 8, 2008, p. 287–313.

7. A. Gibofsky and R.L. Barkin, "Chronic pain of osteoarthritis: Considerations for selecting an extended-release opioid analgesic," *Am J Therapeut,* vol. 15, 2008, p. 241–55.

8. Ibid.

9. J. Manzanares, M. Julian and A. Carrascosa, "Role of the cannabinoid system in pain control and therapeutic implications for the management of acute and chronic pain episodes," *Curr Neuropharmacol,* vol. 4, 2006, p. 239–57.

10. C. Sostres, C.J. Gargallo, M.T. Arroyo et al., "Adverse effects of nonsteroidal anti-inflammatory drugs (NSAIDs, aspirin and coxibs) on upper gastrointestinal tract," *Best Pract Res Clin Gastroenterol,* vol. 24, 2010, p. 121–32.

11. B. Caldwell, S. Aldington, M. Weatherall et al. "Risk of cardiovascular events and celecoxid: A systematic review and meta-analysis," *J R Soc Med,* vol. 99, 2006, p. 132–40; L.C. Chen and D.M. Ashcroft, "Risk of myocardial infarction associated with selective COX-2 inhibitors: Meta-analysis of randomised controlled trials," *Pharmacoepidemiol Drug Saf,* vol. 16, 2007, p. 762–72.

12. S.D. Solomon, J.J. McMurray and M.A. Pfeffer et al., Cardiovascular risk associated with celecoxib in a clinical trial for colorectal adenoma prevention," *Engl J Med,* vol. 352, 2005, p. 1071–80.

13. FDA, "Joint Meeting of the Arthritis Advisory Committee and the Drug Safety and Risk Management Advisory Committee," 16–18 February 2005. [www.fda.gov/ohrms/dockets/ac/05/minutes/2005-4090L1_Final.pdf]; R. Chou, M. Helfand, K. Peterson et al., "Comparative effectiveness and safety of analgesics for osteoarthritis," (Internet), Rockville (MD): Agency for Healthcare Research and Quality (US), 2006. Report No. L06-EHC009-EF. AHRQ Comparative Effectiveness Reviews; J. Witter, "Celebrex capsules (celecoxib) medical officer review," www.fda.gov/ohrms/dockets/ac/01/briefing/3677b1_03_med.pdf.

14. F. Silverstein, L. Simon and G. Faich, "Reporting of 6-month vs. 12-month data in a clinical trial of celecoxib," *JAMA*, vol. 286, 2001, p. 2399–400.

15. A. Inotal and A. Mészáros, "Economic evaluation of nonsteroidal anti-inflammatory drug strategies in rheumatoid arthritis," *Int J Technol Assess Health Care*, vol. 25, 2009, p. 190–95.

16. D.W. Kaufman, J.P. Kelly, L. Rosenberg et al., "Recent patterns of medication use in the ambulatory adult population of the United States: The Slone survey," *JAMA*, vol. 287, 2002, p. 337–44.

17. N.J. Shaheen, R.A. Hansen, D.R. Morgan et al., "The burden of gastrointestinal and liver diseases," *Am J Gastroenterol*, vol. 101, 2006, p. 2128–38.

18. American Geriatrics Society Panel on Pharmacological Management of Persistent Pain in Older Persons, "Pharmacological management of persistent pain in older persons," *J Am Geriat Soc*, vol. 57, 2009, p. 1331–46.

19. C. Sostres, C. J. Gargallo, M.T. Arroyo et al., "Adverse effects of nonsteroidal anti-inflammatory drugs (NSAIDs, aspirin and coxibs) on upper gastrointestinal tract," *Best Pract Res Clin Gastroenterol*, vol. 24, 2010, p. 121–32.

20. American Geriatrics Society Panel on Pharmacological Management of Persistent Pain in Older Persons, "Pharmacological management of persistent pain in older persons," *J Am Geriat Soc*, vol. 57, 2009, p. 1331–46.

21. J.D. Katz and T. Shah, "Persistent pain in the older adult: What should we do now in light of the 2009 American Geriatrics Society Clinical Practice Guideline?" *Pol Arch Med Wewn*, vol. 119, 2009, p. 795–800.

22. D.W. Kaufman, J.P. Kelly, L. Rosenberg et al., "Recent patterns of medication use in the ambulatory adult population of the United States: The Slone survey," *JAMA*, vol. 287, 2002, p. 337–44.

23. S. Staube, M.R. Tramer, R. Andrew Moore et al., "Mortality with upper gastrointestinal bleeding and perforation: Effects of time and NSAID use," *BMC Gastroenterol*, vol. 9, 2009, p. 41–48.

24. J.W.J. Bijlsma, "Patient benefit-risk in arthritis: A rheumatologist's perspective," *Rheumatology* (Oxford), vol. 49 (suppl. 2), 2010, p. iii1–iii17; J. Brun and R. Jones, "Non-steroidal anti-inflammatory drugs-associated dyspepsia: The scale of the problem," *Am J Med,* vol. 110 (1A), 2001, p. 12s–13s.

25. S. Hernández-Dias and L.A. Garcia-Rodriguez, "Association between nonsteroidal anti-inflammatory drugs and upper gastrointestinal tract bleeding/perforation: An overview of epidemiological studies published in the 1990s," *Arch Intern Med,* vol. 160, 2000, p. 2093–99.

26. C. Sostres, C.J. Gargallo, M.T. Arroyo et al., "Adverse effects of nonsteroidal anti-inflammatory drugs (NSAIDs, aspirin and coxibs) on upper gastrointestinal tract," *Best Pract Res Clin Gastroenterol,* vol. 24, 2010, p. 121–32; S. Staube, M.R. Tramer, R. Andrew Moore et al., "Mortality with upper gastrointestinal bleeding and perforation: Effects of time and NSAID use," *BMC Gastroenterol,* vol. 9, 2009, p. 41–48.

27. B. Schlansky and J.H. Hwang, "Prevention of non-steroidal anti-inflammatory drug-induced gastropathy," *J Gastroenterol,* vol. 44, 2009, p. 44–52.

28. Ibid.

29. R. Chou, M. Helfand, K. Peterson et al., "Comparative effectiveness and safety of analgesics for osteoarthritis" (Internet), Rockville (MD): Agency for Healthcare Research and Quality (US), 2006. Report No. L06-EHC009-EF. AHRQ Comparative Effectiveness Reviews.

30. A. Risser, D. Donovan, J. Heintzman et al., "NSAID prescribing precautions," *Am Fam Physician,* vol. 80, 2009, p. 1371–78.

31. J.W.J. Bijlsma, "Patient benefit risk in arthritis: A rheumatologist's perspective," *Rheumatology* (Oxford), vol. 49 (suppl. 2), 2010, p. iii1–iii17.

32. A. Risser, D. Donovan, J. Heintzman et al., "NSAID prescribing precautions," *Am Fam Physician,* vol. 80, 2009, p. 1371–78.

33. Ibid.

34. T.C. Campbell and T.M. Campbell, *Le Rapport Campbell. Révélations stupéfiantes sur les liens entre L'Alimentation et la santé à long terme,* Outremont, Éditions Ariane, 2008, 488 p.

13 ATTEMPTS TO EXPLAIN THE LACK OF CONSENSUS ON USING TARGETED NUTRITION TO PREVENT AND TREAT MANY CHRONIC DISEASES (DESPITE THE PUBLICATION OF NUMEROUS CONVINCING STUDIES)

1. P. Kopelman and J. Lennard-Jones, "Nutrition and patients: A doctor's responsibility," *Clin Med,* vol. 2, 2002, p. 391–94.

2. T.C. Campbell and T.M. Campbell, *Le Rapport Campbell. Révélations stupéfiantes sur les liens entre L'Alimentation et la santé à long terme,* Outremont, Éditions Ariane, 2008, 488 p.

3. Ibid.
4. Ibid.
5. Ibid.
6. Ibid.
7. Ibid.
8. Ibid.
9. M. Angell, "Is academic medicine for sale?" *New Engl J Med,* vol. 342, 2000, p. 1516–18.
10. M. Angell, "Drug Companies and Doctors: A Story of Corruption," *New York Review of Books,* January 15, 2009.
11. T.C. Campbell and T.M. Campbell, *Le Rapport Campbell. Révélations stupéfiantes sur les liens entre L'Alimentation et la santé à long terme,* Outremont, Éditions Ariane, 2008, 488 p.
12. Ibid.
13. R. Maillard, "Marketing sur ordonnance," *Protégez-vous,* mai 2010, p. 8–12; R. Maillard, "La grande manipulation," *Protégez-vous,* mai 2010, p. 18–19.
14. R. Maillard, "Marketing sur ordonnance," *Protégez-vous,* mai 2010, p. 8–12.
15. Ibid.
16. R. Maillard, "La grande manipulation," *Protégez-vous,* mai 2010, p. 18–19.
17. R. Maillard, "Marketing sur ordonnance," *Protégez-vous,* mai 2010, p. 8–12.

EPILOGUE

1. T.C. Campbell and T.M. Campbell, *Le Rapport Campbell. Révélations stupéfiantes sur les liens entre L'Alimentation et la santé à long terme,* Outremont, Éditions Ariane, 2008, 488 p.
2. S. Champagne, "A l'école de la douleur," *La Presse,* July 19, 2010, cahier A.
3. Ibid.

REFERENCES FOR THE FOREWORD

R.D. Altman, "Ibuprofen, acetaminophen and placebo in osteoarthritis of the knee: A six-day double-blind study" [abstract], *Arthritis Rheum,* vol. 42, 1999, S403.

J.P. Case, A.J. Baliunas, J.A. Block, "Lack of efficacy of acetaminophen in treating symptomatic knee osteoarthritis: A randomized, double-blind, placebo-controlled comparison trial with diclofenac sodium," *Arch Intern Med,* vol. 163, 2003; p. 169–78.

J.D. Deeks, L.A. Smith, M.D. Bradley, "Efficacy, tolerability, and upper gastrointestinal safety of celecoxib for treatment of osteoarthritis and rheumatoid arthritis: Systematic review of randomised controlled trials, *Brit Med J,* vol. 325, 2002, p. 619–27.

G.P. Geba, A.L. Weaver, A.B. Polis, M.E. Dixon, T.J. Schnitzer, "Efficacy of rofecoxib, celecoxib, and acetaminophen in osteoarthritis of the knee: A randomized trial," *JAMA,* vol. 287, no. 1, 2002; p. 64–71.

C.G. Helmick, D.T. Felson, R.C. Lawrence et al., "Estimates of the prevalence of arthritis and other rheumatic conditions in the United States. Part I," *Arthritis Rheum,* vol. 58, no. 1, 2008, p. 15–25.

L. Laine, "Nonsteroidal anti-inflammatory drug gastropathy," *Gastrointest Endosc Clin N Am,* vol. 6, no. 3, 1996, p. 489–504.

R.C. Lawrence, D.T. Felson, C.G. Helmick et al., "Estimates of the prevalence of arthritis and other rheumatic conditions in the United States. Part II," *Arthritis Rheum,* vol. 58, no. 1, 2008, p. 26–35.

J. Porter, H. Jick, "Addiction rate in patients treated with narcotics," *N Engl J Med,* vol. 320, 1980, p. 123–26.

G. Singh, O. Wu, P. Langhorne, R. Madhok, "Risk of acute myocardial infarction with nonselective non-steroidal anti-inflammatory drugs: A meta-analysis," *Arthritis Res Ther,* vol. 8, no. 5, 2006, p. 153–62.

S.D. Solomon, J.J. McMurray, M.A. Pfeffer et al., "Cardiovascular risk associated with celecoxib in a clinical trial for colorectal adenoma prevention," *N Engl J Med,* vol. 352, 2005, p. 1071–80.

T.E. Towheed, L. Maxwell, M.G. Judd, M. Catton, M.C. Hochberg, G. Wells, "Acetaminophen for osteoarthritis," *Cochrane Database Syst Rev,* 2006, 1:CD004257.

M. Weaver, S. Schnoll, "Addiction issues in prescribing opioids for chronic nonmalignant pain," *J Addict Med,* vol. 1, no. 1, 2007, p. 2–10.

APPENDIX 1
Characteristics of the small intestine

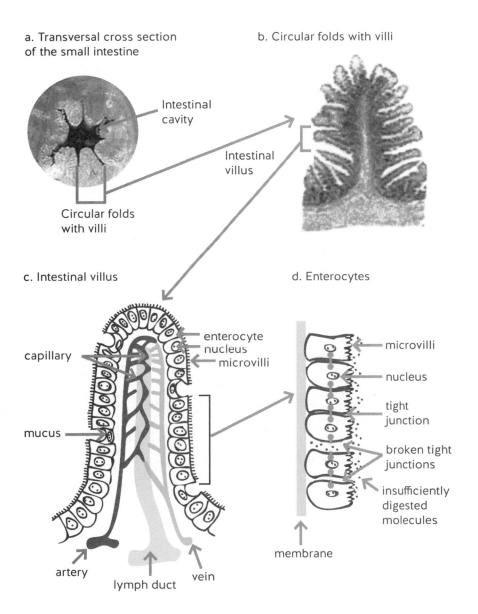

a. Transversal cross section
of the small intestine

b. Circular folds with villi

Intestinal
cavity

Intestinal
villus

Circular folds
with villi

c. Intestinal villus

d. Enterocytes

capillary

enterocyte
nucleus
microvilli

microvilli

nucleus

tight
junction

mucus

broken tight
junctions

insufficiently
digested
molecules

membrane

artery

vein

lymph duct

APPENDIX 2
B lymphocytes are involved in the specific immune response through the production of antibodies

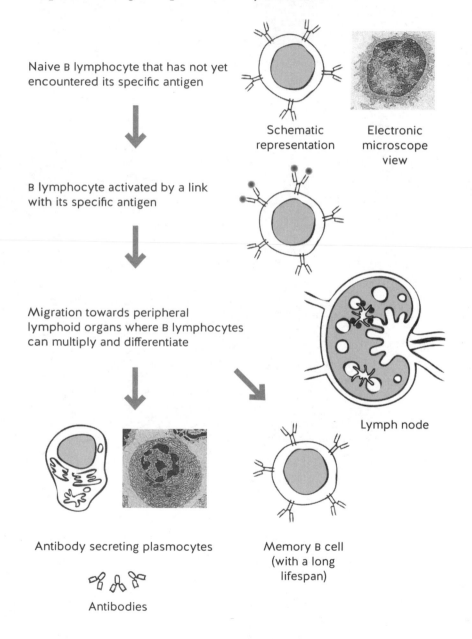

Naive B lymphocyte that has not yet encountered its specific antigen

Schematic representation

Electronic microscope view

B lymphocyte activated by a link with its specific antigen

Migration towards peripheral lymphoid organs where B lymphocytes can multiply and differentiate

Lymph node

Antibody secreting plasmocytes

Antibodies

Memory B cell (with a long lifespan)

APPENDIX 3
T lymphocytes are involved in the cell-specific immune response

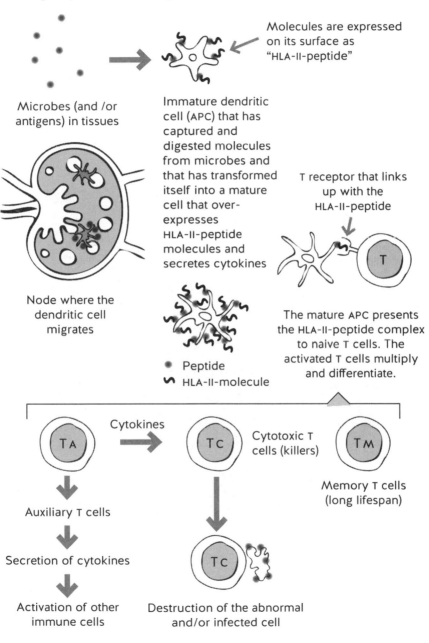

Molecules are expressed on its surface as "HLA-II-peptide"

Microbes (and /or antigens) in tissues

Immature dendritic cell (APC) that has captured and digested molecules from microbes and that has transformed itself into a mature cell that over-expresses HLA-II-peptide molecules and secretes cytokines

T receptor that links up with the HLA-II-peptide

Node where the dendritic cell migrates

• Peptide
∿ HLA-II-molecule

The mature APC presents the HLA-II-peptide complex to naive T cells. The activated T cells multiply and differentiate.

TA — Cytokines → TC — Cytotoxic T cells (killers) — TM

Memory T cells (long lifespan)

Auxiliary T cells

Secretion of cytokines

Activation of other immune cells

Destruction of the abnormal and/or infected cell

APPENDIX 4

Various white blood cells or leukocytes involved in the innate (nonspecific) immune response: Part A

POLYMORPHONUCLEAR:
Neutrophil: Phagocytic activity—they capture, ingest and digest inert and live particles. Bactericide activator.

Eosinophil: They eliminate antibody-coated parasites.

Basophile: Have immunomodulatory action, and play an essential role in inflammation. Could be present in mucus.

MONOCYTE: Precursor cell that transforms into macrophage when it moves from the bloodstream to the tissues.

IMMATURE DENDRITIC CELL: All dendritic cells express HLA-II molecules. They maintain their immature shape as long as their HLA-II molecules are not linked to their complementary antigen.

APPENDIX 5

The various white blood cells or leukocytes involved in the innate (nonspecific) immune response: Part B

These leukocytes are only present in tissues.

MACROPHAGE: A phagocytic cell with an additional role of antigen presenting cell.

MAST CELL: Releases granules containing histamine and serotonin. They are involved in inflammation and hypersensitive reactions.

DENDRITIC CELL: Becomes mature and active in lymph nodes. Captures antigens and presents them to T lymphocytes.

* **DIAPEDESIS:** Enables leukocytes to cross blood capillaries to move into surrounding tissue

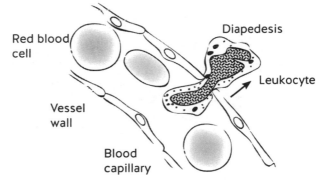

Red blood cell

Diapedesis

Leukocyte

Vessel wall

Blood capillary

* Leukocytes normally present in the bloodstream can pass out of the capillaries by diapedesis to reach infected and/or inflamed tissues.

APPENDIX 6

The role of HLA-I molecules (specific immune response)

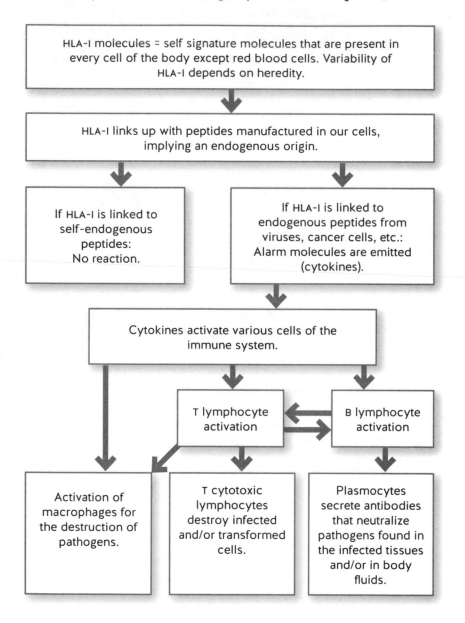

APPENDIX 7
The role of HLA-II *molecules (specific immune response)*

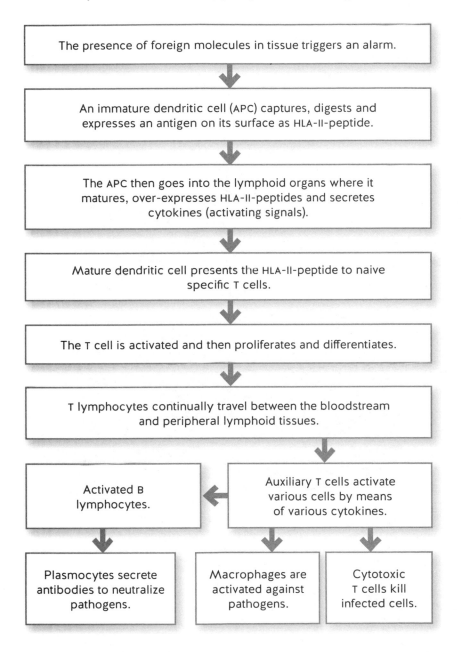

The presence of foreign molecules in tissue triggers an alarm.

An immature dendritic cell (APC) captures, digests and expresses an antigen on its surface as HLA-II-peptide.

The APC then goes into the lymphoid organs where it matures, over-expresses HLA-II-peptides and secretes cytokines (activating signals).

Mature dendritic cell presents the HLA-II-peptide to naive specific T cells.

The T cell is activated and then proliferates and differentiates.

T lymphocytes continually travel between the bloodstream and peripheral lymphoid tissues.

Activated B lymphocytes.

Auxiliary T cells activate various cells by means of various cytokines.

Plasmocytes secrete antibodies to neutralize pathogens.

Macrophages are activated against pathogens.

Cytotoxic T cells kill infected cells.

APPENDIX 8

Hypothesis on the cause of celiac disease:
An autoimmune disease associated with HLA-II molecules, either HLA-DQ2 or -DQ8*

*Note: DQ2 could be replaced by DQ8 anywhere below

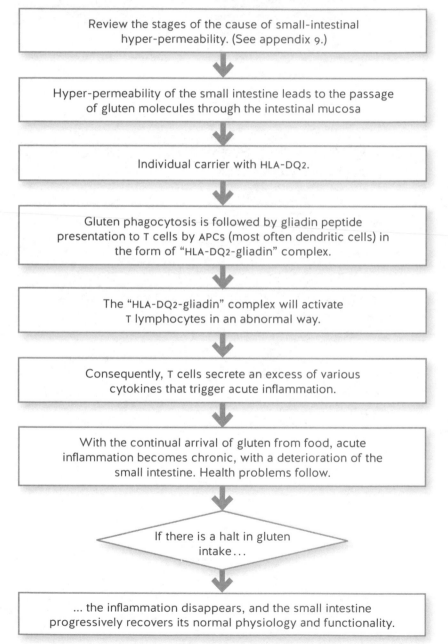

Review the stages of the cause of small-intestinal hyper-permeability. (See appendix 9.)

Hyper-permeability of the small intestine leads to the passage of gluten molecules through the intestinal mucosa

Individual carrier with HLA-DQ2.

Gluten phagocytosis is followed by gliadin peptide presentation to T cells by APCs (most often dendritic cells) in the form of "HLA-DQ2-gliadin" complex.

The "HLA-DQ2-gliadin" complex will activate T lymphocytes in an abnormal way.

Consequently, T cells secrete an excess of various cytokines that trigger acute inflammation.

With the continual arrival of gluten from food, acute inflammation becomes chronic, with a deterioration of the small intestine. Health problems follow.

If there is a halt in gluten intake...

... the inflammation disappears, and the small intestine progressively recovers its normal physiology and functionality.

APPENDIX 9

Causes of hyper-permeability of the small intestine

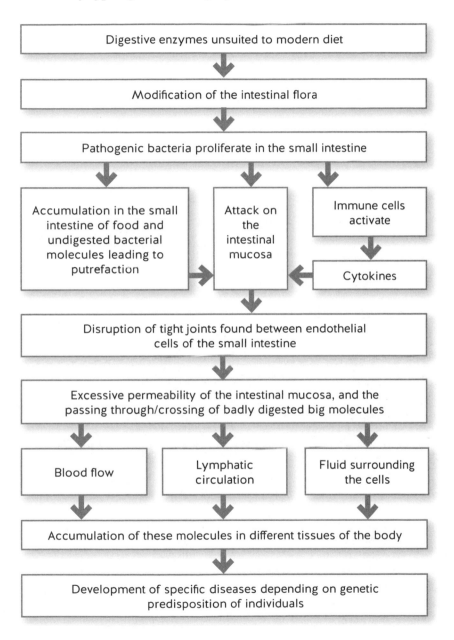

INDEX

acne, 187, 189–90
acrylamide
    American consumption of, 91–92,
        92
    in common foods, 212
    overview, 91–92
    and plant cultivation, 92
    reducing consumption of, 93
    toxicity, 91
    See also glycotoxins
Actimel, 117–18
Activia, 117–18
advanced glycation end-products
    (AGE). *See* glycotoxins
advertising of food, 203, 204
AGE. *See* glycotoxins
alkaline-acid balance, 77–79, 115–16
almonds, 116
Alzheimer's disease, 34, 38, 175
American Geriatrics Society, 198
American Medical Students
    Association, 209
American Psychiatric Association, 207
ancestral diet. *See* hypotoxic diet
ancient diet. *See* prehistoric diet
Angell, Marcia, 205

angiogenesis, 177–78, 179
ankylosing spondylitis, 146, 168–70
antibiotics, 49
antigen-presenting cells. *See* APC
antigens
    altered, 142
    food, 60, 61, 163, 166
    nonself, 142
    self, 142
    See also superantigens
anti-inflammatory medicines, 49
APC, 51, 55, 140, 143, 144–45
apoptosis, 72, 73
arthritis, rheumatoid
    beginning in intestines, 60
    cause, 141
    and celiac disease, 67
    and cereals, 66
    characteristics, 149–50
    cofactors, 33, 149, 151–52, 160
    defined, 60
    diagnostic signs, 150
    and elementary diet, 61
    food's role, 152, 162–67
    genetic predisposition, 20, 61,
        149, 160

HLA molecules, 149
hormones, 160–61
hypotoxic diet, 148–67
and identical twins, 33
inflammatory response, 153–54
and intestinal flora, 60–61
joint lesions, 150–51
meatless diet, 60
medication, 151
Mediterranean diet, 165–66
pathogenesis, 32
recurrence, 159
Seignalet's theory, 152–55, 155–56, 178–79
Seignalet's treatment, 157–59
smoking, 160–62
triggers, 60
twins, 151
and vitamin D, 127
See also arthrosis
arthrosis
angiogenesis, 177–78, 179
cause suggested, 179–80
cause unknown, 177
characteristics, 176–78
current treatments, 176
deposit pathology, 175
halted by diet, 181
hypotoxic diet, 32, 180–81
inflammatory process, 8
pain, 177
Seignalet's theory, 178–79
and supplements, 127, 128–29
wear and tear, 177
See also arthritis, rheumatoid
asparagine, 91, *92,* 104
aspirin, 199
asthma, 33, 70, 190–92
autism, 67–68
autoimmune diseases
cow's milk, 73

gluten, 55–56
HLA, 147
hypotoxic diet, 148, 168–72
modern diet, 40
overview, 145–47
prevalence in the West, 52–53
procedure for treating, 172
table of, *34*
Western diet, 53
autoimmune pathology, 32, 175–76
autoimmune process, halting, 56, 97
autoimmune reactions, 145–46, 147

B lymphocytes, 47, 51, 140, 145, *268*
Bach, Edward, 25
bacterial flora. *See under* small
intestine
basophils, 48, 138, *270*
Baxter Healthcare, 202
Béliveau, Richard, 23
Bextra, 197
Bio-K+, 118–19
bone loss, 76, 81, 126, 127
bone resorption, 79, 82, 115
bovine spongiform encephalopathy,
76
brain, human, 69–70
breastfeeding, 58, 68–69, 69–70,
160–61
Brion, Pierre, 208
Bristol-Myers-Squibb, 202
buckwheat, 104
Burger, Guy-Claude, 26

calcium
daily intake, 123
daily requirements, 81
deficiency, 103
list of foods containing, 80
in mineral water, 114
neutralizes acidity, 116

sources of, 79–80, 103
vitamin D, 125–27
Campbell, Colin T., 166–67, 200, 202, 203–4, 205–6, 210
Canada, dairy-product consumption, 74
"Canada's Food Guide," 81
Canadian Food Inspection Agency, 130
cancer
    breast, 71, 83, 112, 126, 175
    colorectal, 126, 175
    cow's milk, role in, 73
    and hypotoxic diet, 34, 38
    IGF-1 hormone, 71–72
    and meat consumption, 83
    ovarian, 71
    prostate, 71, 112, 175
    RAGES, 94
    uterine, 71
cannabinoids, 195, 196
cardiovascular disease, 69, 83, 112, 125–26, 130, 197, 199
Carton, Paul, 25
cattle-rearing practices, 75–76
Celebrex, 197, 200
celiac disease
    cause, 274
    and cereals, 66
    environmental factors, 51–52
    genetic predisposition, 20, 55–56
    gluten, 20, 55–56, 67
    HLA molecules, 20, 51–52, 55, 274
    onset, 52
    prevalence of, 67
    and tight junctions, 56
    See also gliadin; gluten
cereals
    central to modern diet, 203
    domesticated, 63, 65–68
    elimination of, 211
    harmful effects, 66–68
    and human evolution, 65
    modification of, 65–66
    portion of modern diet, 64
    See also grains
chemotherapy, 50
children
    asthma, 191
    Crohn's disease, 188
    dairy product consumption, 72–74
    intelligence quotient, 70
    and phytoestrogens, 113
    small-intestinal hyper-permeability, 191
chondroitin sulfate, 128–29
chronic disease
    environmental cofactors, 39
    genetic predisposition, 39
    glycotoxins, 86–87
    in hunter-gatherers, non-Westernized societies, 64
    industrialized milk production, 75–76
    insulin secretion, 73
    intestinal integrity, 45
    linked to glycotoxins, 96–98
    onset, 52–62
    pathogenesis of, 31
    prevented by changes in cooking, 95
    result of inflammation, 140
    treatment of, 31
chronic inflammatory disease
    causes, 32
    costs, 214
    diagnosing, 62
    and modern diet, 32, 53
    multifactorial nature, 33
    onset, 52
    three groups of, 148

chyle, 45
cigarettes, 160–61
citrullination, 149–50
cofactors
    food, 20
    gliadin, 20
    rheumatoid arthritis, 33, 149,
        151–52
    triggers of disease, 20
    See also environmental factors
colitis, ulcerative, 53, 54, 70, 187–88
comorbidity, 150, 196, 198
conjunctivitis, 187
conventional medicine
    failure of, 5, 8
    fibromyalgia, 181
    intestinal microflora, 62
    and specialization, 31
cooking of food
    cereals, 66
    and glycotoxins, 87
    hazards of, 82–96
    at high temperatures, 26, 67,
        82–83, 95, 103, 105, 212
    and human diet, 63
    meat, 105
    microwave, 95
    mutagenic effects, 94, 105
    produces glycotoxins, 87, 91,
        165, 212
    reducing hazards of, 94–95
corticosteroids, 195
cow's milk, 49
    and blood insulin levels, 72–73
    compared to breast milk, 68–69,
        69–70
    harmful effects of, 68–82
    human consumption begins, 63
    inflammatory response to, 59
    not suited to humans, 73,
        103–05, 167

origin of chronic disease, 75
and pregnancy, 74
and type 1 diabetes, 73–75
See also dairy products
Crohn's disease, 33, 53, 54, 56, 66, 70,
    187, 188
cytokines, 43, 49–50, 138, 145, *269*
cytotoxic cells. *See* killer T cells

daidzein, 112
dairy products
    acne, 189
    alternatives to (for calcium),
        79–80
    and blood insulin, 72–73
    and calcium deficiency, 103
    central to modern diet, 203
    glycotoxins, 88
    increase in chronic disease, 54
    mineral water as substitute, 114
    osteoporosis, 76–77
    promote disease, 104
    promoted, 80
    type 1 diabetes, 75–76
    unsuited to humans, 211
    See also cow's milk
dairy-free diet, 67–68
Danone, 117–18, 202, 204
Demers, Sylvie, 72
dendritic cells, 48, 51, 137, *270, 271*
deposits
    arthrosis, 176–78
    cause of arthrosis, 179–80
    concept of, 174–75
    diseases of, 34, *35,* 174
    fibromyalgia, 182
    and lifestyle, 184
    Maillard reaction, 179–80
    pathology, 32, 33, 40, 148, 173–85,
        175–76, 178, 179
dermatitis, atopic. *See* acne

dermatitis herpetiformis, 66, 67
diabetes, type 1
    breastfeeding, 70
    calcium and vitamin D, 126
    cereals, 66
    cow`s milk, 73
    dairy products, 75–76
    development of, 71
    fructose, 133
    HLA molecules, 146
    intestinal flora, 57
    intestinal hyper-permeability, 57
    intestinal immunity, 58
    milk consumption, 73–75
    milk production, 76
diabetes, type 2
    deposit pathology, 175
    diagnosis, 183
    fructose, 133
    genetic predisposition, 184
    hypotoxic diet, 32, 184–85
    and meat consumption, 83
    milk consumption, 72
    not insulin dependent, 57
    overview, 182–83
    Seignalet's hypothesis, 183–84
    vitamin D and calcium, 126
*Diagnostic and Statistical Manual of
    Mental Disorders (DSM)*, 207
diapedesis, 139, *271*
Dionne, Jean-Yves, 96
double-blind method, 26–27
drugs. *See* medication

eczema, 67, 187, 190
EFSA, 117–18
elementary diet, 61, 162
Eli Lilly, 204
elimination, diseases of, 34, *36*, 40,
    186–92
elimination pathology, 32, 82–83, 148

End of Pain, 8–9, 22
enterocytes, 43, 44, 45, 46, 47, 49, 153
enteroviruses, 58
environmental factors
    acne, 189
    ankylosing spondylitis, 168–70
    asthma, 191
    celiac disease, 52, 56
    in chronic disease, 39, 53
    diabetes, type 2, 183
    fibromyalgia, 181, 182
    and genetic predisposition, 61
    immune-mediated disease, 98
    multiple sclerosis, 171
    nonself antigens, 97
    rheumatoid arthritis, 160
    subject to change, 156, 210
enzymes
    action of, 41–42
    and digestion, 40–41, 82
    disfunction of, 42
    enemies of, 42
    heredity, 41–42
    and modern foods, 42, 49, 103
    overview of, 40–42
    substrate, 41
eosinophils, 48, 138, *270*
epidemiological studies, to evaluate
    diet, 28–29
epithelium, intestinal, 43, 44
Epstein Barr virus, 161
Esselstyn, Caldwell B., 29, 203
European Food Safety Authority
    (EFSA). *See* EFSA
evolution, human, and diet, 63, 64, 65
excretory organs, 186
exercise, 81

fasting, and rheumatoid arthritis,
    162–63
fats, saturated, 121, 122, 129, 132–33, 203

fats, trans, 13, 121, 129, 130, 131, *132,* 132–33, 203
fatty acids, 122, 129, 131, 132, 133, 165–66
FDA, 125, 130, 197
fibromyalgia, 32, 59–60, 181–82
Finland, dairy-product consumption, 74
food
    acrylamide content, 91–92, *92*
    and body renewal, 39
    and cell function, 39
    cofactor in chronic disease, 20, 33, 39, 53
    emotional ties to, 203
    and enzymes, 40–41
    glycotoxin content, 88, *89, 90*
    micronutrients, 119–23
food, industrial
    changes in human diet, 63
    chronic disease, 85–86
    consequences, 122–23
    effects of, 121
    high-fructose corn syrup, 133–34
    micronutrient decline, 120
    overview, 64
food labeling, 109, 117–18, 121, 130–32, *132*
food synergy, 123–24
food-industry regulation, 121–22
foods, analysis of, 103–07
fractures, hip, 126
fractures, vertebral, 126
Fradin, Jacques, 26
free radicals, 42, 50, 141–42
fructose, 133–36
fruits, 105, 116, 134, 135

Gagnon, Marc-André, 207
gallstones, 34

Gardens for Research, Experiential Education and Nutrition, 120
genetic predisposition
    asthma, 191
    celiac disease, 20, 55–56
    and chronic pain, 20
    diabetes, 184
    and environmental cofactors, 39, 56, 61, 210
    fibromyalgia, 181, 182
    and multiple sclerosis, 170
    rheumatoid arthritis, 61, 149
    and small-intestinal hyper-permeability, 50–52
    See also environmental factors; heredity
genetic sensitivity. *See* genetic predisposition
genistein, 112, 113
gliadin, 20, 51–52, 55, 56, 58
    See also gluten
globalization, and farming, 40
glucosamine sulfate, 128–29
glucose, 134
gluten
    associated diseases, 67
    celiac disease, 20, 67, 96–97, *274*
    intolerance, 49, 55–56, 67–68
    See also gliadin
gluten-free diet, 20, 56, 67–68
glycoproteins, in mucus, 40
glycotoxins
    average consumption, 85
    and chronic disease, 84, 86–87
    in common foods, *89, 90*
    defenses against, 86–87
    foods high in, 88
    and fructose, 134
    increased disease risk, 87
    and life span, 84–86
    linked to chronic disease, 96–98

Maillard reaction, 83
  in meat and cereals, 95
  tissues affected, 87
  See also acrylamide
goitre, 114
Gøtzsche, P., 27, 28
government regulation of food, 93,
  121–22, 203, 215
grains, 103–05, 104
  See also cereals
Graves disease, 146

Hampl, R., 114
Hancock, K.D, 113
Health Canada, 93
Heaney, R. P., 81
heredity, 41–42, 43, 62, 174
  See also genetic predisposition
high-fructose corn syrup (HFCS),
  133–34
Hippocrates, 201
HLA molecules
  autoimmune diseases, 146–47
  autoimmune reactions, 146
  celiac disease, 51–52, 67, *274*
  description, 143
  genetic predisposition, 50–52, 61
  immune response, 144–45
  rheumatoid arthritis, 160
  role, 144–45, *272, 273*
  self and nonself, 50–51, 55–56
  small-intestinal hyper-
    permeability, 50–52
  and superantigens, 155
hormones, 43, 71, 76, 112, 114, 160–61,
  183
Hormones au féminin, 72
Hospital of the University of
  Montreal, 213
Hôtel-Dieu, 213
Hróbjartsson, A., 27, 28

Hunt, C.D., 81
hunter-gatherers, 40, 62, 63, 64, 65
hypertension, 126, 133
hypothyroidism, 114
hypotoxic diet
  arthrosis, 180–81
  autoimmune diseases, 168–72
  basic principles, 100–11
  benefits and requirements, 100–03
  clinical testing, 32
  colitis and irritable bowel, 188
  development of, 6
  deviations from, 21, 110–11
  diabetes, 184–85
  differences from other ancestral-
    type diets, 211
  diseases responding to, 34–37
  and double-blind method, 26
  early tests, 26
  effects on intestine, 184
  failures, 33, 38, 158, 169–70, 172,
    180, 182, 185, 188, 190, 192
  fibromyalgia, 182
  key elements, 39–99
  Lagacé's experience of, 21
  lifetime commitment, 21, 158, 185
  mechanism, 159
  and placebo effect, 27, 28
  primary objective, 101
  remission, not cure, 20, 185
  rheumatoid arthritis, 148–67
  rules, 156–57
  successes, 33, 34, 158–59, 169–70,
    172, 180, 182, 185, 188, 190, 192
  theory and observations, 31–34

IGF-1 hormone, 71–72
immune response
  B and T lymphocytes, 140
  bacteria, 173–74
  cytokines, 145

HLA molecules, 144–45
innate, 57, 140
and intestinal bacteria, 62
and leukocytes, 48
molecular mimicry, 61, 155, 166, 171
and nonself antigens, 96
specific, 138, 140
superantigens, 155–56
and tight junctions, 45
immune system
adaptive, 57, 97, 138–39
errors, 51
innate, 97, 137, 138, 183, *271*
intestinal, 159
specific (*see* adaptive)
strategies, 137–47
immune tolerance, 48, 194
industrialized agriculture, 40, 63
inflammation
acne, 189
beneficial, 194
chronic, 140
of excretory organs, 187
as immune response, 138
obesity, 183
subclinical, 140
inflammatory responses
acute, 139
chronic, 140–42
and diet, 141–42
overview, 137–39
rheumatoid arthritis, 153–54
insulin levels, 72
International Diabetes Federation, 183
intestinal flora, 58, 59–60, 60–61
intestinal germs, 54
intestinal immunity, 58–59
irritable bowel syndrome, 59–60, 67, 187–88
isoflavones, 112–13

Janeway, C.A., 137
Japan, and diet, 53–55, 74, 114
Johnson & Johnson, 204
Johnson, L.K., 81

kidney disease, and fructose, 135–36
killer T cells, 48, *269*
Kousmine, Catherine, 25, 94, 115, 171
Kraft, 204

lactic acid bacteria. *See* probiotics
Lagacé, Jacqueline
background, 9
begins hypotoxic diet, 13
chronic pain, 11–16
diet's role in her pain, 17–18
discovers Seignalet's work, 18
end of pain, 19, 111
experience with hypotoxic diet, 6–8, 18–22, 21, 107–11, 213
review of scientific literature, 9, 22, 213
uses nutrition therapy, 11–16
L'Alimentation ou la troisième médecine, 8, 18, 33, 148
"leaky gut." *See* small-intestinal hyper-permeability
legumes, 80, 102, 103, 105, 116
L'Epicerie, 93
leukemia, 175
leukocytes, 47–48, *270, 271*
life span, and glycotoxin ingestion, 84–86
lifestyle, and disease, 122, 183–84, 201, 214

macrophages, 51, 137, *271*
macular degeneration, 128
mad cow disease, 76
Maillard reaction
acrylamide, 91

AGE, 83
chronic-disease pathology, 84
deposits, 179–80
described, 82
as disease trigger, 98
glycotoxins, 211–12
mutagenic effects, 94
small-intestinal hyper-
    permeability, 82
whole wheat bread, 103
Maillard, Rémi, 206
major histocompatibility complex
    (MHC), 50, 149
margarines, 130, 131
marketing, of medication, 206–7
mast cells, 44, 48, 137, *271*
Mayer, A.N., 119–20
McCance and Widdowson, 119–20
McDonald's, 204
meat, 40, 54–55, 105, 116, 121
medical establishment, 29, 201–9,
    203, 213
medication
    anti-inflammatory, 193–94
    diabetes, 183
    disappointing results, 189
    fibromyalgia, 181
    inefficient, 156
    for inflammatory disease, 193–200
    as late intervention, 156
    non-recommended use, 208–9
    not a cure, 191
    overconsumption, 122
    rheumatoid arthritis, 151
    risks, 199
    side effects, 198–200, 208–9
Mediterranean diet, 28, 80, 101–02,
    165–66
Melnik, B.C., 70, 73, 74
memory T cells, 48, 145, *269*
menopause, 76, 77, 79, 112–13, 125, 126

mental health, and micronutrient
    deficiency, 121
Merck, 209
metabolic acidosis, 77–79, 116, 134, 211
metabolic syndrome, 126, 136
metabolism, and wastes, 39
micronutrients, 119–23, 122, 123–24
microvilli, 45
migraines, 49, 66, 67
milk products. *See* dairy products
mineral water, 82, 114–15
modern diet
    arthritis, 178–79
    bacterial proliferation, 154
    as cause of deposits, 176
    colitis and irritable bowel, 187
    compared to preindustrial diet,
        122
    contrast with prehistoric diet, 40,
        62–64
    disrupts homeostasis, 62
    human enzymes unadapted to,
        42, 64
    and inflammatory disease, 32
    and osteoporosis, 77–79
    putrefaction flora, 116, 173
    and small intestine, 39
    small-intestinal hyper-
        permeability, 188
molecular mimicry, 61, 155, 166, 171
monocyte, *270*
mucus, 44
multiple sclerosis, 66, 170–72
myocardial infarction, 34, 38

National Cattlemen's Beef
    Association, 202
National Dairy Council, 202
National Institutes of Health (NIH),
    205–6
Neolithic Era, 62–64

Nestle Nutrition Institute, 202
Neurotin, 208
neutrophils, 48, 138, *270*
New England Journal of Medicine, 205
NIH, 124
noninflammatory arthritis. *See*
     arthrosis
nonself, 20, 50–51, 96, 142–43, 144,
     152
     See also self
nonsteroidal anti-inflammatory drugs
     (NSAIDS). *See* NSAIDS
NSAIDS, 2, 170, 176, 196–200
nutritherapy. *See* nutrition therapy
nutrition therapy
     alternative to conventional
          medicine, 22–23
     chronic inflammatory disease, 5
     healthcare professionals, 9, 22–23
     lack of training in, 202
     and medical establishment, 201–9
     opposition to, 202–3
     as preventive treatment, 214
     remission of disease, 22–23
     treats disease, 166

obesity, 83, 135, 182–83
oils, 106–07, 164
oligo elements, 123
opioids, 195–96
optimal diet, 210
osteoarthritis. *See* arthrosis
osteoporosis, 76–77, 81–82, 112, 125–
     26, 175
otitis, 187
oxidative stress, 142

pain
     arthrosis, 177
     elimination of, 23
     Lagacé's experience, 11–16

mechanism of, 194
     opioids, 195–96
     remission of through diet, 22–23
painkillers, 193–94, 195
Paleolithic diet, 101–03
Paleolithic Era, 62–64
Paneth cells, 44
parathyroid hormone, 127
Parkinson's disease, 175
Paul, W.E., 137
peanuts, 124
peptides, 144, 152, 155, *269*
peristalsis, 45
pesticides, 50
Pfizer, 204
pH level, 42, 77–78, 79, 115–16
phagocytosis, 139
pharmaceutical industry
     influence of, 203–4, 206–8,
          207–10
     painkillers, 193
     and supplements, 124
PharmFree, 209
physiological balance, 112–37
phytoestrogens, 113
placebo effect, 26–28
polymorphonuclear group, 48,
     137–38, 140, *270*
Portégez-vous, 206, 208
prednisolone, 60, 61
prehistoric diet, 40, 62–64
Prescribe, 207
Prexige, 197
Prim'Holstein cow, 75
probiotics
     bacterial content, 117
     Bio-K+, 118–19
     as capsules, 118
     mechanism of, 117
     overview, 116–19
Proteus mirabilis, 153, 161

pshychosis, 200
psoriasis, 33, 187
psychosis, 67

radiotherapy, 50
RAGE, 84, 94, 98, 212
receptor for advanced glycation end-
    products (RAGE). See RAGE
remission, and hypotoxic diet, 20, 23
research, 204–6, 207–8
rheumatoid arthritis. See arthritis,
    rheumatoid
rice, 104
Royal College of Physicians, 202

schizophrenia, 66
Seignalet diet. See hypotoxic diet
Seignalet, Jean
    acne hypothesis, 189
    on animal proteins, 116
    ankylosing spondylitis
        hypothesis, 169
    on arthrosis, 176
    arthrosis theory, 178–79
    asthma theory, 191
    attempts to publish work, 26
    on autoimmune diseases, 145–46
    background, 5–6, 24–25, 31
    on cooking, 82–83, 98, 105, 211
    deposition hypothesis, 33,
        173–85
    develops hypotoxic diet, 6, 25
    diabetes (type 2) hypothesis,
        183–84
    elimination theory, 186–87
    on enzymes, 41, 42
    epidemiological studies, 28
    funding problems, 28
    on grains, 103
    greatest achievement, 20, 25
    hypotoxic diet as remission, 20

    influences on, 25–26
    on margarine, 130
    on multiple sclerosis, 170–71
    and nutrition therapy, 5, 24
    revised theories, 33
    rheumatoid arthritis theory, 32,
        152–55, 155–56
    on small-intestinal hyper-
        permeability, 49, 61
    success with hypotoxic diet, 6
    on supplements, 123
    tests hypotoxic diet, 26
    treats acne, 190
    treats ankylosing spondylitis,
        169–70
    treats asthma, 192
    treats colitis and irritable bowel,
        187–88
    treats Crohn's disease, 188
    treats eczema, 190
    treats fibromyalgia, 182
    treats multiple sclerosis, 171–72
    treats rheumatoid arthritis, 148,
        157–59
    treats type 2 diabetes, 184–85
    work unknown, 8
    See also hypotoxic diet
selenium, 123
self, 20, 50–51, 142–43, 144
    See also nonself
seniors
    NSAIDS, 198, 199, 200
    painkillers, 196
    and probiotics, 117
    and vitamin D, 126
sinusitis, 187
small intestine
    bacterial flora, 45–47, 55, 57, 156
    characteristics, 267
    defenses, 47–48
    main functions, 44–45

small-intestinal hyper-permeability
    and autoimmune disease, 57
    causes, 49–50, *275*
    chronic disease onset, 52–62
    consequences, 52
    genetic predisposition, 50–52
    overview, 48–49
    pediatric Crohn's disease, 188
    in pediatric disease, 191
    rheumatoid arthritis, 153
    See also small-intestinal
        permeability; tight
        junctions
small-intestinal permeability
    and bacteria, 46, 55
    in children, 48
    development, 40
    and enzymes, 42
    See also small-intestinal hyper-
        permeability; tight
        junctions
small-intestine integrity, 43–52, 45
smoking, 160–61
soil, and micronutrients, 120
soy, 112–14
soy milk, 113
sporadic ataxia, 67
stress, 122
substrate, and enzymes, 41
sugars, 106, 133–36, 134
superantigens, 154, 155–56
    See also antigens
supplements, 123–29

T lymphocytes, 48, 51–52, 56, 144–45,
    155, *269*
targeted diet. *See* nutrition therapy
testimonials, 29–31, 213
testosterone, 113
The Chemical Composition of Foods, 120
Thomas, D., 119–20

Thomas, David, 120
tight junctions, *267*
    arthritis, 179
    in chronic disease development,
        97
    early theory about, 96
    and intestinal integrity, 45
    and onset of inflammatory
        disease, 52
    role, 43–44, 47
    as weakest link, 49
    See also small-intestinal hyper-
        permeability;
        small-intestinal permeability
tinnitus, 200
tolerance and autoimmunity, 142–43
tolerance, oral, 159
Tornqvist, Margareta, 91
trace elements, 123
Trock, B.J., 112
Tylenol, 12, 15, 16, 129

United Dairy Industry Association,
    204–6
United States Department of
    Agriculture, 29
uric acid, and fructose, 135
U.S. Food and Drug Administration.
    See FDA
U.S. National Academy of Sciences,
    131
U.S. National Institutes of Health
    (NIH). *See* NIH

Vadeboncoeur, Alain, 207–8
Vase, Riley and Price analysis, 27
vegetables, 105, 116
villi, intestinal, 43, *267*
Vioxx, 194, 197, 200, 209
vitamin A, 127–28
vitamin C, 127–28, 142

vitamin D, 125–27
vitamin E, 127–28, 142
Vlassara, H., 83

Western diet
    abundant in glycotoxins, 85
    and acrylamide, 91
    causes excess acidity, 77–78, 115
    compared with prehistoric diet,
        63–64
    increases autoimmune diseases, 53
    and the Inuit, 83
    and Japanese study, 54
    linked to inflammation, 122
    and salt, 79

Women's Health Initiative, 71–72
World Congress on Pain, 213
Wyeth-Ayerst, 202
Wylde, Bryce, 3

yogurt, 19, 103, 105, 109, 117, 118, 119

Zaffran, Marc, 206
zonulin, 96, 97